THE OXFORD BOOK OF
HEALTH FOODS

The late J.G. Vaughan (1926–2005) was a botanist and food scientist, and Emeritus Professor of Food Sciences at King's College London. He wrote many books on botany and food plants, among them the widely acclaimed *New Oxford Book of Food Plants* (1997).

P.A. Judd is Professor of Nutrition and Dietetics at the University of Central Lancashire. She has undertaken research and published on various aspects of applied nutrition and dietetics and has a special interest in functional foods and the health claims made for foods and their constituents.

THE OXFORD BOOK OF
HEALTH FOODS

J. G. VAUGHAN & P. A. JUDD

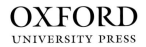

OXFORD

UNIVERSITY PRESS

OXFORD

UNIVERSITY PRESS

Great Clarendon Street, Oxford OX2 6DP

Oxford University Press is a department of the University of Oxford.
It furthers the University's objective of excellence in research, scholarship,
and education by publishing worldwide in

Oxford   New York

Auckland   Cape Town   Dar es Salaam   Hong Kong   Karachi
Kuala Lumpur   Madrid   Melbourne   Mexico City   Nairobi
New Delhi   Shanghai   Taipei   Toronto

With offices in

Argentina   Austria   Brazil   Chile   Czech Republic   France   Greece
Guatemala   Hungary   Italy   Japan   Poland   Portugal   Singapore
South Korea   Switzerland   Thailand   Turkey   Ukraine   Vietnam

Oxford is a registered trade mark of Oxford University Press
in the UK and in certain other countries

Published in the United States
by Oxford University Press Inc., New York

© Oxford University Press, 2003

British Library Cataloging in Publication Data
Data available

Library of Congress Cataloging in Publication Data
Data available

Typeset by Pantek Arts Ltd, Maidstone, Kent
Printed on acid-free paper by
Lito Terrazzi s.r.l., Italy

ISBN 0-19-280680-7 978-0-19-280680-2
1 3 5 7 9 10 8 6 4 2

This book is dedicated to the memory of Professor Arnold Bender – an outstanding nutritionist, food scientist, and educator.

Foreword

When I decided to read Botany back in the early Fifties, most universities had departments dedicated to the subject and all budding students of medicine had to have at least an A-level qualification in biology. This provided them with knowledge of the evolution of their species and the *materia medica*: the basis of the vast majority of the drugs and medicines that they would one day prescribe to their patients. Lowson's *Textbook of botany* was the bible that linked their profession with the heritage of over 60 000 years of herbal health care that they accessed through their local pharmacist, who turned hand-written prescriptions into healing pills, tisanes, and powders.

Despite the Flower Power Sixties all that has changed, so much so that there are few if any departments of Botany *sensu stricto* left to choose from. What is more, as so-called complementary medicine is now all the rage, mainstream medics are less able to counsel their patients as to the efficacy of the plants that still provide at least the green-print of a vast array of proprietary brands on sale in pharmacies today – let alone about the potential interactions between the new mainstream medicines and the food they eat, much of which is tainted with novel agricultural chemicals.

This superb book from the Oxford stable links us all back to that heritage through a vital selection of the so-called health foods now available to the public. The link is not only in the text but in the superb illustrations, some of which take you back to the great herbal texts of the past, while some make your mouth water, reminding us of the fact that Hippocrates himself not only produced the oath of ethical practice but also counselled humankind with the words 'Let your food be your medicine and your medicine be your food.'

The text elegantly sets out the heritage mix of botany, folklore, and hard scientific fact that is now coming to the fore, as an ever-wider cross section of people is demanding access to herbal medicine and healthier lifestyles, and as the pharmaceutical industry, high street outlets, and an increasing number of farmers markets, do their best to keep up with the demand.

David Bellamy
Bedburn, October 2002

Preface

From earliest times there has been a strong connection between food and medicine.

Let your food be your medicine and your medicine be your food.

Hippocrates

In relatively recent years there has been a profusion of so-called 'health foods' that are sold in health food shops and other outlets. These items range from products that are usually regarded as straightforward foods to supplements of possible therapeutic value.

This book constitutes an overview of health foods – the part they play in our diet and their contribution to health and wellbeing. As far as is possible, and when it is available, the scientific basis of these functions is discussed.

A very large number of items may be classified as health foods. In the present work it has not been possible to deal with all of them. However, those that are described are a representative selection of items available in commercial outlets.

The amount of relevant literature, in the form of books, research papers, the Internet, magazines, and others, is very great. In this work, a list of references for further reading is given; these will provide much more information for the interested reader.

The sources of illustrations in this book are recorded elsewhere, but in addition, paintings of many of the food plants referred to are found in *The new Oxford book of food plants* by J.G. Vaughan and C.A. Geissler.

It is important to emphasize that any reader wishing to use a herbal remedy should consult a physician or qualified health professional regarding its efficacy, side-effects, and interactions with other drugs. Similarly, those who buy food products for health reasons should consult a state-registered dietitian or reputable nutritionist.

In this book, medical and scientific terms have been kept to a minimum and a glossary is included to explain the terms we regarded as essential.

This book should be of interest to biologists, physicians, nutritionists, dietitians, other health professionals, as well as the many members of the public who utilize health foods.

Acknowledgements & sources of figures

ACKNOWLEDGEMENTS
We acknowledge with many thanks the assistance given by the following: Dr H. Prendergast, S. Davis, Frances Cook, Susyn Andrews, Dr G. Lewis, Marilyn Ward, Chris Leon, Professor Monique Simmonds, Dr Madeleine Harley, Dr M. Nesbitt (Royal Botanic Gardens, Kew); Dr D. Bender (University College London); Professor Varro E. Tyler (USA); Professor P. Houghton, Dr Amala Raman, A. Howard, Professor H. Baum, Dr Peter Ellis, Professor Jeremy Mason (King's College London); UK Health Food Association; Dr Barbara Steinhoff (Germany); Bee Health Ltd (UK); Pharma Nord Ltd (UK); Dr R.A. Hughes (St Peter's Hospital); Dr B. Jones, Dr J. Blackshaw (Food Standards Agency); Dr G. Rodger (Marlow Foods, UK); Statfold Seed Oils Ltd (UK); A. Chevallier; P. York (Natural History Museum, London); C.W. Lut (Leiden); Dr S.R. Hoskins; R. Macmillan.

We would also like to thank the staff of Oxford University Press for editorial and technical guidance, and Liz Moor for typing the manuscript.

SOURCES OF FIGURES
Bentley, R. and Trimen, H. (1880). *Medicinal plants.* London.
Aloe, Senna, Slippery elm

Bernard Thornton Artists.
Alfalfa, Artichoke, Bamboo, Chickweed, Cranberry, Echinacea, Evening primrose, Ginseng, Hawthorn, Henna, Meadowsweet, Nettle, Orris, Parsley piert, Pineapples, Skullcap, Thuja

Epple, A.O. (1995). *A field guide to the plants of Arizona.* Helena, Montana, USA.
Jojoba

Harden, Gwen J. (ed.) (1991). *Flora of New South Wales.* Vol. 2. Sydney.
Tea tree

Hayne, F.G. (1805). *Getreue Darstellung und Beschreibung der in der Arzneykunde Gebrauchlichen gewächse.* Berlin.
Astragalus, Bilberry, Borage, Burdock, Carob, Celery seed, Roman chamomile, Drosera, Eyebright, Garlic, Horsetail, Hyssop, Milk thistle, Motherwort, Pilewort, Plantain, Pulsatilla, Rose hip, St John's wort, Strawberry, White bryony, White willow

King's College London.
Hemp, New Zealand mussel, Pulses, Pumpkin, Sesame, Soya bean, Sunflower

Kohler's *Medizinal-Pflanzen* (1887). Leipzig.
Angelica, Arnica, Balm, Buchu, Cayenne pepper, Centaury, German chamomile, Coltsfoot, Comfrey, Dandelion, Deadly nightshade, Elder, Fennel, Feverfew, Ginger, Goldenseal, Guarana, Holy thistle, Hops, Ipecacuanha, Laminaria (seaweed), Lavender, Lime, Linseed, Liquorice, Lobelia, Lycopodium, Marigold, Marshmallow, Mistletoe, Peppermint, Quassia, Raspberry, Rue, Sage, Sumach, Sweet flag, Sweet violet, Uva-ursi, Valerian, Witch hazel, Yarrow

Marlow Foods, Stokesley, UK.
'Quorn'

Nationaal Herbarium Nederland, Leiden, The Netherlands.
Californian poppy, Ginkgo, Wild yam

Natural History Museum, London, UK.
***Spirulina* (algae)**

Royal Botanic Gardens, Kew, UK.
Pollen: dandelion and mallow

Thompson, W.A.R. (ed.) (1978). *Healing plants.* London.
Damiana, Devil's claw, Kava kava, Saw palmetto, Wild yam

Contents

Contents

Introduction

The term 'health food' is used to describe a whole range of foods and dietary supplements commonly sold in health food shops.

The supplements range from essential nutrients, such as vitamins and minerals in varying doses, through to those that might best be described as herbal remedies. When considering foodstuffs, calling them health foods is perhaps unfortunate as it carries the implication that other foods are inherently unhealthy. This is of course not the case, but products sold in health food stores are often seen to have some sort of additional benefits beyond the consumption of a healthy, balanced diet. This book aims to examine systematically some of the foods and products sold under the health food banner and show where there is evidence for benefit from the wide range of products available.

Current nutritional thinking is that most foods can be eaten as part of a healthy diet as long as the balance of foods is right. The converse of this is that if the diet is balanced and eaten in the right amounts to satisfy a person's energy needs, that person will also obtain all the nutrients he or she requires. Government expert committees strive to determine what the nutrient requirements might be for all sections of the population, and most countries produce guidelines for both the balance of nutrients such as protein, fat, and carbohydrate, and recommended daily intakes for micronutrients such as vitamins and minerals. However, some people believe that the recommended intake levels do not take sufficient account of individual requirements, which will vary according to genetic make-up, stage of life,

life-style, and possibly physical and emotional stresses. The concept of 'optimal nutrition' or 'nutritional medicine' has therefore been proposed, whereby individuals may seek to improve aspects of their life and health by supplementing their diets in various ways. The 'orthodox' view is often that nutritional supplements are unnecessary and that it is better to achieve the required amount by eating foods containing them. This also ensures that any as-yet unknown potentially beneficial food components are also consumed. However, this may not always be possible, and certain sections of the public may benefit from supplementation in some circumstances.

Dietary supplements may take the form of vitamins, minerals, and trace elements, or plant extracts, which, although not generally regarded as nutrients are now recognized to have potential health benefits. Certain foods may also be seen as having particular health benefits. Some, such as soya, naturally contain a variety of potentially beneficial materials; others, such as yoghurts containing probiotic bacteria, or margarine with added plant sterols, are manufactured to have particular benefits. These latter products are sometimes called functional foods or nutraceuticals. Some of them have been subjected to extensive scientific research and have proven benefits; for others the situation is less clear-cut, and the following pages will attempt to indicate when this is so.

In order to make best use of the information in the book some background about nutrition and herbal medicine is given here.

Nutrition

ENERGY

In order to live and carry out all daily activities we need energy. Most of the energy supplied by our food and drink is used to maintain basic body functions, i.e. it keeps the heart beating, the blood circulating, and the lungs and other major organs, including the brain, constantly working. A variable amount of energy is needed in addition to the basal metabolism to account for activity – for most people this adds up to half as much as the basal requirement to the day's needs. Energy is measured in kilocalories (kcal) or kilojoules (kJ) (1 kcal is 4.18 kJ). Although scientists use the precise term kcal, most people simply call this unit a 'calorie', and adults generally require between

1500 and 3000 kcal or calories per day to maintain body weight, depending on gender, body size, and activity level. Taking in more energy than required (or not compensating for a high energy intake by increasing activity) results in weight gain; insufficient energy intake for the level of activity you do results in weight loss.

Energy is supplied by the major components of our food, i.e. carbohydrate, fats, and protein (sometimes called macronutrients), as well as by alcohol. One gram of pure carbohydrate or protein provides approximately 4 kcal, while fat supplies 9 kcal per gram and alcohol 7 kcal per gram; however, as few foods are composed of just one nutrient, the energy content of the food depends largely

Introduction

on the amount of water in the food and the proportions of protein, fat, and carbohydrate (including dietary fibre) making up the dry weight. For example, foods such as fruits and vegetables generally contain large amounts of water, no fat, little protein, and varying amounts of carbohydrate, but because of the high water content may have energy values as low as 1 kcal per gram, whereas foods with a high fat and low water content, such as nuts, will have energy values in excess of 6 kcal per gram.

Dietary fibre, or non-starch polysaccharides (see below), are considered to be part of the carbohydrate component of foods but supply about 2 kcal per gram. A high dietary fibre content therefore acts to dilute the energy content of a food.

CARBOHYDRATES

Carbohydrates are the main source of energy for most populations throughout the world. Plant foods supply most of the carbohydrates eaten by adults since most foods of animal origin contain negligible amounts. The exception to this is lactose, or milk sugar, an important energy source for babies but less important in the adult diet. Dietary carbohydrates range from simple sugars to complex molecules such as starches or non-starch polysaccharides, and are classified according to the number and configuration of the single sugar units (monosaccharides) joined together. Simple sugars – the monosaccharides and disaccharides – are sweet, and foods containing these are often seen as particularly palatable because of this.

Monosaccharides

All carbohydrates are made up of carbon, hydrogen, and oxygen, and depending on the number of carbon atoms in the backbone may be trioses (3C), tetroses (4C), pentoses (5C), hexoses (6C), or heptoses (7C). The most important dietary carbohydrates are the 5 and 6 carbon sugars – the pentoses and hexoses. Some of these exist as monosaccharides but more commonly are found joined as chains of various lengths. Glucose is a hexose, and the main form in which carbohydrate is absorbed into the bloodstream. It is rarely found free in natural foods (small amounts in some fruits and vegetables), although some occurs in honey. Fructose is found in honey, fruits, and some vegetables. Another hexose, galactose, is a characteristic component of lactose or milk sugar, and also a common component of some of the complex storage carbohydrates in plants such as legumes. Pentose sugars such as ribose and deoxyribose are components of deoxyribonucleic acid (DNA) and ribonucleic acid (RNA), and so are present in minute amounts in all foods.

Disaccharides

These are combinations of two simple sugars. Sucrose, a combination of glucose and fructose, is the most common disaccharide; extracted from sugar cane and sugar beet, it is present naturally in some fruits and vegetables. Other common disaccharides are lactose – the sugar found in milk (glucose and galactose) – and maltose (glucose plus glucose), which is formed when barley sprouts during the brewing process. Malt extracts and malted milk drinks will contain maltose.

Oligosaccharides

Oligosaccharides are short chains of sugars with three to nine sugar molecules. The most common of these (raffinose, stachyose, and verbascose) are found in legumes and are not digested by human digestive enzymes – they are digested by bacteria in the large intestine, producing gas. Fructo-oligosaccharides (FOS), especially inulin, found in Jerusalem artichokes, and others found in onions, garlic and some cereals, have recently drawn interest as they appear to function as prebiotics (see later), encouraging the growth of particular, supposedly beneficial bacteria – the so-called probiotics – in the large intestine.

Polysaccharides

This group of carbohydrates covers a wide range of compounds all containing long chains of sugar molecules joined together. They may contain only one type of sugar e.g. starch. Starches are the major polysaccharide and carbohydrate in the human diet, and contain only glucose. Others – the non-starch polysaccharides – usually contain at least two different sugars and may contain several different types. For example, there might be a backbone of one type of sugar such as galactose, with side chains of another, e.g. mannose – such a compound would be called a galactomannan. There are many different types of non-starch polysaccharides, depending on the plant source and the function within the plant. Cellulose is a common non-starch polysaccharide, and non-cellulosic polysaccharides such as pectins, and plant gums such as gum arabic and guar gum, are other examples.

The way in which the molecules are joined together affects their structure and properties. There are different types of linkages between the sugar molecules that may result in the compound being a straight chain or having branches. The types of linkages also affect their availability to human digestive enzymes. Starch is made up of two types of chains of glucose molecules: amylose is an unbranched form while amylopectin is highly branched.

Introduction

Starches from different plant sources differ in the proportions of amylose and amylopectin, and this also affects the availability of the glucose from the starch in the food, especially after cooking and cooling. Raw starch is indigestible, and must be cooked with some water in order to gelatinize it and make it available to the amylase enzymes in the gut.

Digestion and absorption of carbohydrates

A small amount of digestion of cooked starch commences in the mouth where there is a salivary amylase, but carbohydrates are mainly digested in the small intestine by enzymes (alpha amylases) secreted by the pancreas and also present in the wall of the intestine. The resultant monosaccharides are absorbed into the bloodstream and carbohydrate absorption can be tracked by measuring blood glucose levels at intervals after a meal. The blood glucose level rises rapidly for the first 30 minutes or so after a meal and returns to baseline in about 2 hours as it is taken into tissues under the influence of insulin and other hormones. It is now recognized that the rate of rise in blood glucose and subsequent fall to baseline levels (glycaemic response) is not the same for different sources of carbohydrates. Many factors influence this; these include: (a) whether the carbohydrate is given as a simple solution such as glucose, or in a more complex food form; (b) the relative proportions of amylose and amylopectin in a starchy food; (c) the presence of non-starch polysaccharides in the food; (d) the form of the food, e.g. finely ground versus large particles of grain; (e) the cooking method; and (f) the presence of other nutrients in the food, e.g. fat.

Extensive trials have compared the glycaemic response to different carbohydrate sources, and the concept of the glycaemic index has been developed. The glycaemic index predicts the rate at which blood glucose will rise after a particular food compared with the rate at which it would rise after an equivalent amount of white bread. If the glycaemic index of white bread is taken as 100, then wholemeal bread is 52, white spaghetti 32, sucrose 58, baked beans 48, and soya beans 18. These indices are especially useful if incorporated into the diet of people with diabetes mellitus, where it is important to control the levels of blood glucose between defined limits in order to prevent complications. Low glycaemic index diets can help to achieve this.

Non-starch polysaccharides are generally not digested by the human amylases because the enzymes cannot break the beta linkages between the molecules, and are part of what has more commonly been known as dietary fibre.

Dietary fibre

Dietary fibre has been defined as the plant materials that are resistant to the human digestive enzymes. Dietary fibre includes non-starch polysaccharides, as described above, but the early methods for measuring the dietary fibre content of foods also resulted in the inclusion of non-carbohydrate materials such as lignin (the woody part of plants), cutins, and waxes as well as some resistant starch (see below). Although the term dietary fibre is now well understood by the public, scientists investigating the potential beneficial effects of the complex prefer to be more precise and refer only to the specific non-starch polysaccharides, ignoring the resistant starch, lignins, and other materials.

This has resulted in some confusion over the dietary fibre content of foodstuffs, as some countries (and even sometimes within countries) use total dietary fibre, and others non-starch polysaccharides, as the measurement on food labels and in food composition tables. The use of non-starch polysaccharides results in apparently lower levels of 'unavailable' material in the foods, as can be seen from the British food composition tables where both values are recorded.

Different foods contain different types of non-starch polysaccharides and this may have different effects on health. For example, cellulose and other non-starch polysaccharides from cereals are less fermentable by gut bacteria than the so-called soluble non-starch polysaccharides found in foods such as oats and some fruits and vegetables. The former may be beneficial in terms of preventing constipation and some bowel diseases, whereas the latter, such as the beta-glucans in oats or guar gum from the cluster bean (*Cyamopsis tetragonoloba*), may help lower blood cholesterol levels and modulate blood glucose levels. Foods containing fibre supplements of various types are now being marketed as 'health foods' or 'functional foods'.

Resistant starch

It used to be thought that all starch in foods was digested and absorbed, but it is now recognized that a certain proportion of the starch in foods is not digested in the small intestine and therefore enters the large intestine, along with the non-starch polysaccharides in the diet, where fermentation by gut bacteria breaks the materials down. Starch is resistant to digestion for various reasons. It may be enclosed within grains, which if not broken down by chewing survive the upper intestine intact; the structure of the starch grains within the food may resist digestion; reheating and subsequent cooling of the food may have resulted in the formation of retrograded starch whose

Introduction

structure again resists the action of amylase; or the processing method itself may affect the structure of the starch. Whatever the reason, starch is probably the most important substrate for fermentation, greater even than the non-starch polysaccharides – simply because it is present in larger amounts.

Fermentation by bacteria results in the production of a variety of gaseous materials as well as water. Some of these materials are thought to help maintain the health of the large intestine (butyrate), others are absorbed and enter the energy systems of the body (acetate, propionate), while yet others are excreted as wind.

FAT

Fats and oils are the most energy dense component of foods, supplying 9 kcal per gram of the pure substance. Because of this high energy density fat supplies 40% or more of the energy in the diet in many developed countries, although in some developing countries, mainly reliant on plant sources for their energy, the proportion may be as low as 10%. Chemically, fats and oils are lipids, defined as substances that are insoluble in water, but soluble in organic solvents such as alcohol. Fats are usually solid at room temperature, e.g. butter or lard, while oils are liquid but very similar chemically.

As well as triglycerides, which make up the main part of dietary fat, lipid materials include such things as sterols and phospholipids. Lipids are very important in the body; as well as providing an energy store (triglycerides), they are important in maintaining the structure of cell membranes, and sterols such as cholesterol also provide the basis for a wide range of hormones, including the reproductive hormones. Phospholipids are important because they are miscible in both lipids and water and act to stabilize emulsions. For example, in the body they help to maintain cell membrane structure, and in foods lecithins, found naturally in egg yolk, peanuts, and soya, are used to stabilize foods such as chocolate and mayonnaise.

Although fats and oils have generally similar structures, there are differences that are important to health. In the diet the most important fats and oils are triglycerides, whose chemical structure consists of three fatty acid molecules attached to a molecule of glycerol. Fatty acids are composed of chains of carbon atoms of varying length, with hydrogen atoms attached at the bonding sites. Depending on how many hydrogen atoms are attached at each carbon bond, the fatty acids may be termed saturated or unsaturated. If sites are saturated there is a single bond between the carbon atoms, and where sites are unsaturated a double bond occurs.

Fatty acids are therefore classified according to the length of the carbon chain and the number of double bonds.

- Short chain fatty acids have 4–6 carbon atoms, medium chain 8–12, long chain 14–18, and very long chain 20 or more.
- Saturated fatty acids have no double bond, monounsaturated fatty acids have one, and polyunsaturated fatty acids have several double bonds.

The longer the chain length of the constituent fatty acids and the more saturated these are, the harder the fat. Thus lard contains a high proportion of saturated fatty acids, corn oil contains a high proportion of long-chain polyunsaturated fatty acids, and fish oils contain very-long-chain polyunsaturated fatty acids

Unsaturated fatty acids may exist in two distinct forms, *cis* or *trans*. The *trans* form is less common in natural fats but is produced during processing, e.g. in the manufacture of margarines. High intakes of *trans* polyunsaturated fatty acids, it has been suggested, act in a similar way to saturated fatty acids in their effects on blood cholesterol levels.

A further complication in the chemistry of unsaturated fatty acids is that they exist in three different 'families', according to the position of the first double bond in the molecule. Thus fatty acids may belong to the n-3, n-6, or n-9 family. Humans can insert a double bond at position 9 but not at positions 3 or 6. The diet must therefore include some n-3 and n-6 fatty acids, and these are termed the essential fatty acids and sometimes also called omega-3 and omega-6 fatty acids. Recommendations from organizations such as the Food and Agriculture Organization and the World Health Organization are that linoleic acid (n-6) should supply 4–10% and linolenic acid (n-3) 0.5–4% of dietary energy, with a ratio of 0.1:0.4 for n-3:n-6.

Fats and oils in foods contain mixtures of fatty acids. Plant foods contain fats with mainly polyunsaturated fatty acids (40–60%) and monounsaturated fatty acids (30–40%), with up to about 20% of saturated fats. In animal fats the greatest proportion are saturated fatty acids (40–60%), with some monounsaturated fatty acids (30–50%) and less polyunsaturated fatty acids (approximately 10%). There are exceptions to all rules, and some plant fats such as palm oil and coconut oil contain large amounts of saturated fats, while poultry and game tend to have higher proportions of polyunsaturated fatty acids.

Fats and health

Fats are a concentrated source of energy in the diet, supplying 9 kcal per gram no matter what the composition of

Introduction

the constituent fatty acids. Thus for many developed populations where food is plentiful and activity levels not as great as they might be, high-fat, energy-dense, palatable foods may contribute to weight gain. However, at the opposite end of the scale low-fat diets (less than 10% energy from fat) may result in malnutrition if given to young children, as such diets are bulky and the child may simply not be able to eat enough to satisfy energy requirements. A certain amount of fat is needed to supply the essential fatty acids and also to allow absorption of fat-soluble vitamins A, D, and E – it has therefore been suggested that the levels of fat in the adult diet should not fall below 20% of the total energy intake.

Epidemiological evidence has suggested that high fat intakes, especially saturated fatty acids, are associated with a higher incidence of atherosclerosis (hardening of the arteries) and coronary heart disease. In population studies there is an association between serum cholesterol levels and coronary heart disease death rates. Cholesterol in the blood exists in several forms, the most important being carried in the blood on low-density lipoproteins and high-density lipoproteins. These are therefore usually referred to as low-density lipoprotein cholesterol and high-density lipoprotein cholesterol, respectively. Total cholesterol is the sum of these two types (plus a little very low-density lipoprotein cholesterol). High saturated fat intakes correlate with higher serum cholesterol levels, especially the low-density lipoprotein type. In general saturated fatty acids raise serum low-density lipoprotein cholesterol, polyunsaturated fatty acids lower it, and monounsaturated fatty acids have little effect. However, consumption of monounsaturated fatty acids appears to maintain levels of high-density lipoprotein cholesterol, which removes cholesterol from the arteries and helps protect against coronary heart disease. It is thought that the process of atherosclerosis begins with the oxidation of low-density lipoprotein cholesterol by free radicals; this is then taken into the lining of the arteries by scavenger cells which form lipid-loaded cells called 'foam cells' that accumulate cholesterol and form fatty streaks, narrowing the arteries. The role of polyunsaturated and monounsaturated fatty acids in the formation of these streaks is still controversial. However, recent research suggests that if polyunsaturated fatty acids form part of the cell membranes this may render the low-density lipoprotein cholesterol more susceptible to oxidation, whereas monounsaturated fatty acids appear to convey a protective effect. Fats containing monounsaturated fatty acids may also have beneficial effects by reducing platelet aggrega-

tion, which is important in the production of the blood clots that block the arteries in coronary heart disease. Coronary heart disease is a complex multifactorial disease, and other factors besides dietary fat intake will be important. The presence of antioxidants in the diet and adequate intakes of certain B vitamins (folate and B_{12}) may also be important, but at present most authorities advise reduction of total fat to less than 30% of energy, with 10% or less from saturated fatty acids and polyunsaturated fatty acids, and the remainder made up from foods supplying monounsaturated fatty acids. Fish oils containing very long chain n-3 fatty acids eicosapentaenoic acid and docosahexaenoic acid appear to have a protective effect against coronary heart disease. Recommendations to consume two portions per week of oily fish such as mackerel, salmon, and herring are therefore included in government guidelines to prevent coronary heart disease. These fatty acids are also available as dietary supplements and will be discussed later.

High dietary fat intakes have also been associated with some cancers, e.g. post-menopausal breast cancer, prostate cancer, and bowel cancer, but it is difficult to dissociate the effects of fat from the effects of obesity. However, the guidelines for the prevention of heart disease are probably also applicable to the prevention of cancer.

Dietary cholesterol intake is much less important in raising cholesterol levels than saturated fat – cholesterol is an essential part of cell membranes and is also important in the production of hormones and emulsifying agents in the body. Dietary intake represents about 10% of the amount produced daily in the body. However, when low saturated fat diets are recommended, these will result in lower consumption of cholesterol as the high-fat animal foods containing it will be restricted.

PROTEINS

Proteins are the main nitrogen-containing constituents of animal and plant tissues. They are essential for the synthesis of body tissues and regulatory proteins such as enzymes and hormones. Dietary protein usually accounts for about 10–20% of the energy in human diets. The majority of people in developed populations eat far more protein than is required for the essential functions such as replacing body tissues, and much of the protein is broken down to produce energy.

Proteins are made of selected amino acids from the 20 different amino acids present in nature, and joined together through peptide links (amino group of one protein to acid group of the next) to form an almost infinite

Introduction

number of proteins with different structures and functions. Different combinations and sequences of the polypeptide chains allow them to take up different shapes and carry out particular functions within the organism. Unlike the constituents of carbohydrates and fats, amino acids contain nitrogen as well as hydrogen, carbon, and oxygen, and some also contain phosphorus or sulphur. Eight of the amino acids are essential in adults, i.e. they cannot be made in human tissues and must be obtained from the diet. These are phenylalanine, tryptophan, leucine, isoleucine, valine, threonine, methionine, and lysine. In addition, arginine and histidine are regarded as essential in infants as they cannot make enough for their requirements. The remaining amino acids are non-essential as they can be made in the body.

When proteins in foods are ingested they are digested in the stomach and small intestine, and the constituent amino aids or short peptide chains are then absorbed into the blood, to be carried to tissues where they will be used to manufacture body proteins or non-protein products (e.g. nucleic acids), hormones (e.g. thyroxine), neurotransmitters (e.g. serotonin), or oxidized to provide energy.

Protein quality and intakes

Food proteins do not all have the same capacity to provide nitrogen and essential amino acids to the body. The usefulness or quality of a protein depends on the balance of amino acids and the digestibility of the protein. The body requires particular amounts of each essential amino acid, and an ideal food protein would have an amino acid pattern as close to this as possible. Amino acids that are not part of the required pattern will be used for energy. Animal proteins, especially egg and milk proteins, have amino acid patterns similar to the body's requirements and are used as reference proteins. Plant proteins are relatively low in certain amino acids, and that which is present in the lowest amount relative to requirements is called the limiting amino acid. Methionine and cysteine are the limiting amino acids in legumes, and lysine is the limiting amino acid in cereals. As most populations eat a mixture of proteins this is not usually important – a meal such as beans on toast would correct the deficiencies of both the above food groups. However, if total food intake is too low to satisfy energy requirements, or consists largely of a particular food with a low protein content, protein deficiency may occur.

People in developed countries eating a range of foods that supply sufficient energy are unlikely to be short of protein. Most people eat more than enough, and any protein that is not used to build tissues is used to provide energy. There is therefore no advantage to eating a very high-protein diet. Some athletes take high-protein supplements or specific amino acid supplements, and these will be discussed later.

ALCOHOL

Alcohol is the fourth potential contributor to an individual's energy intake. Most societies have found a way to ferment the carbohydrates in their staple or commonly grown foods to produce an alcoholic drink. Thus beer and whisky are made from barley, rum from sugar, vodka from potatoes, and wine from grapes. Alcohol itself provides little but energy – 7 kcal per gram of pure alcohol consumed, but some alcoholic drinks such as wine and beer may have some health benefits due to antioxidant compounds found in the drink. It has therefore been suggested that moderate consumption of alcoholic drinks protects against coronary heart disease.

MINERALS AND TRACE ELEMENTS

These are a range of inorganic materials that are needed in the body in amounts ranging from relatively large to minute, but all must be supplied by the diet. Calcium, phosphorus, and magnesium are needed in quite large amounts (hundreds of milligrams per day) as they all have structural functions in the bones and teeth. Sodium and potassium, the so-called electrolytes, are also present in quite large amounts in the body, and together with chloride are important in controlling the balance of fluids in the tissues, as well as having other metabolic functions. Iron is sometimes classified as a mineral and sometimes as a trace element (it is needed in milligram amounts each day) and, with the other trace elements, has important effects in maintaining various functions in the body (see Table 1).

Comments regarding some of the important minerals and trace elements follow.

Calcium

Calcium is important not only as the main mineral in bones and teeth but also because it has many other metabolic functions in the body. In developed countries we obtain most of our calcium from milk, and dairy products such as yoghurt. In the UK calcium is added to white flour to replace that taken out by milling. Cereals and green vegetables, as well as small fish bones, also supply useful amounts of calcium, and water supplies sometimes contain significant amounts. Absorption of calcium is dependent on adequate supplies of vitamin D, which is

Introduction

Table 1 Minerals and trace elements: sources, functions, and recommended intakes

Mineral	Dietary sources	Main functions	UK adult RNI[a]	USA adult RDA[a]
Calcium (Ca); also see text	Dairy products: cheese, milk, yoghurt. Bread and breakfast cereals. Fish eaten with bones, e.g. canned sardines, salmon, whitebait. Green, leafy vegetables. Pulses, e.g. baked beans, lentils.	Building and maintenance of the skeleton (and teeth).	700 mg.	1000 mg.[b] Aged 51–70: 1200 mg.
Phosphorus (P)	Milk and milk products, eggs, nuts, cereals, meat and meat products, vegetables, potatoes. Carbonated drinks.	Present in all cells of the body – 85% in skeleton. Important in energy transfer in the body. Dietary deficiency unlikely.	555 mg. Lactation 995 mg.	700 mg.[b]
Magnesium (Mg)	Bread and cereals, beverages, such as beer and coffee, vegetables and potatoes, milk and milk products, meat and meat products.	Linked with Ca in bone development, protein synthesis. Part of many enzyme systems, e.g. in energy transfer.	Males 300 mg, females 270 mg.	Males 400–20 mg, females 310–20 mg. Pregnancy 350–60 mg.
Sodium (Na)	Salt added to food at table or in processing. Concentrated in foods such as ham, bacon, cheese, foods canned in brine, salted nuts, potato crisps or biscuits, yeast extracts, bottled sauces. Bread and breakfast cereals, meat and meat products, and milk also contain significant amounts.	Regulation of fluid balance and blood pressure. Na intakes are usually higher than desirable in developed countries.	1600–2400 mg per day. Average UK intake 3600 mg.	No RDA.
Potassium (K)	Vegetables and potatoes, fruit, drinks, e.g. coffee (especially instant), milk and milk products, chocolate, cocoa, malted milk, yeast extracts, chutneys and pickles, cereals, meat and meat products.	Regulation of acid–alkali balance and fluid balance. Muscle and nerve function. (95% of body's K is present in cells, and total body K is used to measure lean body mass.)	3500 mg.	No RDA.
Iron (Fe) (Also see text)	Meat and meat products. Main source in UK diet is cereals and cereal products because fortified with Fe, followed by meat and then vegetables.	Oxygen carrier in blood and muscle, Enzyme systems for energy transfer. Dietary deficiency possible in women of childbearing age, especially adolescents; infants over 6 months and toddlers; people consuming unbalanced vegetarian diets.	Males 8.7 mg, females 14.8 mg.	Males and post-menopausal females 8 mg. Females of childbearing age 18 mg, pregnancy 27 mg.

continued

Introduction

Table 1 *continued*

Mineral	Dietary sources	Main functions	UK adult RNI	USA adult RDA
Zinc (Zn)	Red meat, fish and shellfish, milk and dairy products, poultry, eggs. Cereals and bread, green leafy vegetables, and pulses are also good sources, but bioavailability is lower compared with animal sources.	Important in many enzyme systems in the body and takes part in metabolism of protein, fat, and carbohydrate. Component of insulin and growth hormone. Subclinical deficiency may occur when requirements are high but intake is reduced due to poor appetite; e.g. postsurgery or infection. Also possible if no animal products eaten and consumption of phytate-containing cereals is high.	Males 9.5 mg, females 7.0 mg. Lactation: extra needed.	Males 11 mg, females 8 mg. Pregnancy 11 mg, lactation 12 mg.
Copper (Cu)	Rich sources are shellfish, liver, nuts, and cocoa. Main sources in UK diet are meat and meat products, cereals, vegetables and potatoes, beverages, e.g. tea and coffee.	Component of a variety of enzymes; contributes to elasticity of collagen and elastin, especially in blood vessels. Involved in antioxidant mechanisms in the body and in prevention of infection.	1.2 mg. Lactation: extra needed.	0.9 mg. Pregnancy 1.0 mg, lactation 1.3 mg.
Chromium (Cr)	Data are not very reliable but good sources thought to be brewer's yeast, meat, wholegrains, legumes, nuts.	Involved in glucose metabolism in form of organic complex known as 'glucose tolerance factor'. Also plays part in protein and fat metabolism.	No RNI; 25 μg is a safe and adequate intake.	Males 35 μg, females 20–5 μg. Pregnancy 30 μg, lactation 45 μg.
Selenium (Se)	Meats, cereals, vegetables, and fats in UK. Depends on Se content of soils, so in USA and Canada cereals will be a better source. Toxic in large amounts. Recommended upper limit from all sources 450 μg.	Antioxidant mineral – glutathione peroxidase, an enzyme that protects tissues from oxidative breakdown, contains Se. May also be involved in protein, fat metabolism, and in thyroid function.	Males 75 μg, females 60 μg. Lactation 75 μg.	55 μg. Pregnancy and lactation 60–70 μg.
Iodine (I)	Milk, seafoods, and dried seaweeds. Iodized salt.	Essential component of thyroid hormones that regulate metabolism. In fetus and infant, protein synthesis in brain and central nervous system is dependent on iodine. Deficiency is rare in Europe and the USA, but is still a problem in many parts of the world.	140 μg.	150 μg. Pregnancy 220 μg, lactation 290 μg.
Fluorine (F)	Water, especially in tea.	Bones and teeth.	No RNI. Water fluoridated at 1 p.p.m.[c] to prevent caries.	Males 4 mg, females 3 mg.

[a]RNI, reference nutrient intake (per day); RDA, recommended daily allowance.

[b]For ages 25–50. For ages 11–25, the recommendation is 1200 mg per day.

[c]p.p.m., parts per million.

Introduction

made in the body in response to exposure to sunshine, but it is also affected by the availability of the calcium in the foods. Calcium in foods forms complexes with other constituents, from which it must be released prior to absorption. These include proteins, oxalates, and possibly the most important, phytic acid phosphorus (usually known as phytate). Phytates in cereal brans and some pulses and nuts bind with the calcium and make it unavailable. When yeast is used in bread-making an enzyme present in the yeast (a phytase) releases the calcium for absorption, but in countries where unleavened wholegrain breads are the staple diet absorption of calcium and other minerals such as iron and zinc is reduced.

Dietary intakes in the UK and USA vary between about 500 and 1200 mg per day, but the proportion of calcium absorbed varies at different stages of the lifecycle according to individual needs. Absorption is highest in infants, during the growth spurt at adolescence, and in pregnancy. Adequate calcium intake is particularly important in the period of growth between onset of adolescence and 18 years of age, as it will affect peak bone mass. This is the maximum amount of bone achieved (mostly laid down by age 18, although small amounts may accumulate up till age 30) and will therefore influence the amount of calcium available to be lost when the process is reversed in later life. A high peak bone mass reduces the likelihood of developing osteoporosis in later life, so calcium intake and weight-bearing exercise in adolescence are very important.

There does not seem to be a need for an increase in calcium intake in pregnancy or lactation. In pregnancy more efficient absorption covers the fetus' requirement. However, during breast-feeding there does not seem to be an increase in absorption, and much of the calcium excreted in the milk comes from the skeleton and by reductions in the amount of calcium excreted in the urine. When the baby is weaned hormonal changes in the woman result in increased absorption, low excretion, and restoration of bone calcium, and there does not seem to be a relationship between lactation and later osteoporosis. The calcium content of breast milk does not seem to be affected by calcium intake.

Rickets in children (and osteomalacia in adults) and osteoporosis are disorders related to bone metabolism. Although low calcium intakes in childhood may result in poor growth, calcium deficiency does not cause rickets or osteomalacia, which are related more to lack of vitamin D. Osteoporosis, which results from the progressive reduction in bone density from middle age onwards, also does not

appear to be related to calcium deficiency at this point in life. Inactivity and the hormonal changes (low levels of oestrogen in women and testosterone in men) accelerate loss of calcium from bone from middle age and a high peak bone mass protects the individual from these effects. Adequate calcium and vitamin D, plus exercise during the years from adolescence to 30, are therefore the most important factors in preventing osteoporosis.

High calcium intakes, whether as food or as supplements, taken at the same meal as foods containing iron will inhibit the absorption of iron from both animal and vegetable sources. This is important, as calcium supplements may be taken by women of child-bearing age, to enable them to achieve peak bone mass, who may have difficulties achieving their necessary level of iron intake and absorption anyway. It may be sensible to monitor iron status in such women. There does not seem to be the same inhibitory effect if calcium and iron are taken together without food. Except in a few people with 'idiopathic hypercalciuria' who absorb excessive amounts of calcium, high intakes do not appear to contribute to the formation of kidney stones because there is a reduction in the amount of calcium absorbed. Intakes above 2500 mg per day as supplements, however, have resulted in cases of milk-alkali syndrome, with high levels of blood calcium, kidney problems, and severe alterations in metabolism.

Iron

The most important role of iron in the body is as an oxygen carrier, in haemoglobin in the red blood cells and myoglobin in muscles. Oxygen is needed for many processes in the body, and is picked up in the lungs by the haemoglobin in the blood flowing through them and carried to the tissues where it is needed. However, iron also has many other functions in the body as part of enzyme systems involved in the transfer of energy between cells and in amino acid metabolism. Too much free iron in the body could be dangerous, and the absorption, transport, and storage of iron in the body are closely regulated. Surplus iron is stored in the liver, spleen, and bone marrow as ferritin (which is readily available when needed) and haemosiderin (an insoluble form).

Iron deficiency is more common than iron overload and is usually due to loss of blood at a rate greater than that at which it can be absorbed from the diet. In developed countries deficiency is most common in women due to heavy menstrual losses, but in developing countries it may be due to infection with intestinal parasites, and affects both men and women. In the UK there is evidence

Introduction

to suggest that low iron intakes are common in women, with most reporting intakes lower than the recommended nutrient intakes. There is a clear association between these low intakes and low haemoglobin and ferritin levels.

Iron is present in the diet in two forms: haem iron in meat and non-haem iron (inorganic salts) in plants. Haem iron is absorbed most efficiently, but if animal products are present in the diet they also seem to enhance non-haem iron absorption, possibly due to the presence of specific amino acids. The absorption of non-haem iron is also facilitated by having a source of vitamin C at the same meal – orange juice with the cereal at breakfast, for example – and by some organic acids. Dietary fibre and phytates associated with this hinder absorption of iron, as do concurrent high calcium intakes and tea. People in groups with a high risk of iron deficiency could possibly maximize absorption of iron by not drinking tea or milk at mealtimes.

VITAMINS

These are substances that are needed in very small amounts each day to maintain normal metabolism. The term 'vitamin' comes from 'vital amines', coined by Dr Casimir Funk in 1913 when these essential nutrients were first discovered. Nutritionists at the beginning of the twentieth century had identified the major nutrients, i.e. carbohydrates, fats, and proteins, and recognized that several mineral elements were also essential for health. However, when animals were fed on diets containing purified mixtures of the known nutrients they failed to grow. This was remedied by adding small amounts of milk to the diets, and further studies identified two factors in the milk. One, called A, was found in the cream and the second, called B, in the watery part of the milk. Factor B was identified as an amine – hence the name. As other different essential substances were identified it became apparent that these were not all amines, and the final 'e' was removed from the name.

The naming of the vitamins was originally alphabetical, i.e. A, B, C, D, and E, but as chemical techniques became more sophisticated it was discovered that vitamin B was a mixture of substances with different functions, and the B vitamins were also given numbers, i.e. B_1, B_2, B_6, and B_{12}. Gaps in the letter sequence relate to substances that were given numbers but later found not to be essential, or substances such as nicotinic acid (niacin) that had already been identified by a specific name and later discovered to be chemically the same as one of the B vitamins. Vitamin F turned out not to be a vitamin, vitamin G was the same as vitamin B_2 and vitamin H is known as biotin – another B vitamin. The alphabetical sequence ends with H; vitamin K is not named in order of discovery but from the Danish term 'koagulation', relating to the function in the blood.

The vitamins are by definition essential, and it was originally thought that they could not be made in the body. This is true for all but two of the vitamins, vitamin D and niacin, originally described as one of the B vitamins. Vitamin D is made in the skin when it is exposed to sunlight and is therefore now considered to be a hormone, but it is essential if sunlight exposure is inadequate, e.g. in housebound people or for those who cover their skin for cultural reasons. Niacin is made in the body from the essential amino acid tryptophan, and deficiency is unlikely to occur except in very particular circumstances.

Vitamins are classified as fat soluble (A, D, E, and K) or water soluble (B vitamins and C). They have a wide range of functions in the body according to their structure and chemistry (see Table 2). Obvious deficiency diseases are rare in developed countries but subclinical deficiencies can occur under certain circumstances, as shown in Table 3.

Table 2 Characteristics of fat-soluble and water-soluble vitamins

	Water-soluble vitamins	Fat-soluble vitamins
Storage in the body	Generally low; require small intakes frequently	May be large and long term
Stability in foods	Variable; may be destroyed by heat or light, or dissolved out during cooking	Generally stable to heat and light
Risk of deficiency	Diets lacking variety	Very low-fat diets – 10% of energy in the diet must be from fat to ensure that they are absorbed; conditions where fat absorption is impaired
Risk of toxicity	Low, as high intakes usually excreted in urine	High

Introduction

Table 3 Vitamins in the diet: sources, functions, recommended intakes, and results of deficiency

	Dietary sources	Main functions and effects of deficiency	UK adult RNI	USA adult RDA
Fat-soluble vitamins				
A As retinol As beta-carotene	Animal foods, including milk, eggs meat. Oily fish and fish liver oils. Green and red vegetables and fruits.	Normal development and differentiation of tissues. *Deficiency*: impaired night vision, loss of integrity of skin and mucous membranes, increased risk of infection. *Toxicity*: liver damage, deformities in fetus if high doses when pregnant.	Males 700μg,[a] females 600μg. Pregnancy 700μg, lactation 950μg. Maximum intake for males: 9000μg, females 7500μg.	Males 900μg, females 700μg. Pregnancy 770μg, lactation 1300μg.
D (calciferol)[b]	Margarines and fat spreads, oily fish, eggs, dairy products. In the UK fortified cereal products provide significant amounts. NB: dietary sources are less important than the 'vitamin' which is made in the skin when exposed to sunlight.	Active form of the vitamin is involved in calcium metabolism. *Deficiency*: rickets in children, osteomalacia in adults.	None unless housebound. Pregnancy, lactation, and aged 65+: 10μg.	Aged 25–50: 5μg; 51–70: 10μg; 71+: 15μg.
E (tocopherols, tocotrienols)	Widespread in foods, mostly from fats as spreads or oils, or in processed foods. Meat, fish, eggs.	Antioxidant – prevents damage to lipid-containing structures in the body, such as cell membranes. *Deficiency*: rare, but possibility that low intakes increase risk of some chronic diseases, such as coronary heart disease and cataracts.	Depends on amount of PUFA[c] in the diet; 0.4mg per g of PUFA suggested.	15mg. Lactation 19mg.
K K1 (phylloquinone) K2 (menaquinone)	K1: green leafy vegetables, soya oil, beef liver, dried seaweed. K2: made by bacteria in the gut.	Blood clotting. *Deficiency*: rare, but results in prolonged clotting time. Infants are born with very low levels, and as the gut is sterile they cannot manufacture vitamin K. An injection is therefore given shortly after birth.	No RNI.	Males 120μg, females 90μg.
Water-soluble vitamins				
B_1 (thiamin)	Bread and cereals, especially wholegrain or fortified breakfast cereals. Potatoes and vegetables, meat and dairy products.	Metabolism of carbohydrates, fats, and alcohol. Requirements related to energy intake. *Deficiency*: most likely to occur in alcoholics: nerve damage. Severe: beriberi.	Males 1.0mg, females 0.8mg.	Males 1.2mg, females 1.1mg. Pregnancy 1.4mg, lactation 1.5mg.

continued

Table 3 *continued*

	Dietary sources	Main functions and effects of deficiency	UK adult RNI[a]	USA adult RDA[a]
B$_2$ (riboflavin)	Rich sources: yeast and yeast extracts, vegetables. Also milk and dairy products, meat, cereals, drinks, especially beer.	Metabolism of carbohydrate and fat-energy production. *Deficiency*: cracks, sores around mouth and nose. Poor B$_2$ status seen in elderly with limited diets.	Males 1.3 mg, females 1.1 mg.	Males 1.3 mg, females 1.1 mg. Pregnancy 1.4 mg, lactation 1.6 mg.
Biotin	Widespread. Rich sources are liver and kidney, yeast, nuts, eggs, pulses, wholegrain cereals. Beer and coffee may provide significant amounts.	Co-factor for enzyme systems in fat metabolism. *Deficiency*: unlikely. Stored in liver.	No RNI. Safe and adequate intake is 10–200 µg.	30 µg. Lactation 35 µg.
B$_6$ (pyridoxine)	Widely distributed in foods. Rich sources: meat, wholegrain cereals, bananas, nuts, pulses.	Metabolism of proteins, carbohydrate, and fats. *Deficiency*: rare, but may occur in alcoholics, and due to interactions with drugs. *Toxicity*: can cause nerve damage at high intakes. High doses sometimes taken to relieve premenstrual syndrome.	Males 1.4 mg, females 1.2 mg. Recommended upper intake 10 mg.	Males 1.2–1.5 mg, females 1.3–1.5 mg. Pregnancy 2.6 mg, lactation 2.8 mg.
B$_{12}$ (cobalamin)	Animal foods only. Rich source: liver.	Functions in range of enzyme systems. *Deficiency*: pernicious anaemia. B$_{12}$ is stored in the liver, and dietary deficiency occurs only in people eating vegan or macrobiotic diets without any fortified foods. Reduced absorption occurs in older people due to lack of intrinsic factor.	1.5 µg. Lactation 2.0 µg.	2.4 µg. Pregnancy 2.6 µg, lactation 2.8 µg.
Niacin (nicotinic acid, nicotinamide)	Meat and fish, wholegrain cereals, yeast extracts, bread and breakfast cereals, milk and dairy products. Also synthesized in the body from the amino acid tryptophan (60 mg tryptophan converts to 1 mg niacin equivalent).	Involved in energy metabolism. *Deficiency*: unlikely as long as adequate protein intake. Pellagra in deprived populations where maize is staple food.	As niacin equivalents. Males 17 mg, females 13 mg. Lactation 15 mg.	As niacin equivalents. Males 16 mg, females 14 mg. Pregnancy 18 mg, lactation 17 mg.
Folate (folic acid)	Rich sources: liver, yeast extract, green leafy vegetables, pulses, oranges. Fortified breakfast cereals (folic acid) important source in UK diet.	Important in cell division. *Deficiency*: most likely to occur in disease states, e.g. malabsorption or leukaemia, and due to interactions with certain drugs. Insufficient intake in the first 12 weeks of pregnancy can result in neural tube defects.	200 µg. Women who may become pregnant should take an extra 400 µg as a supplement.	400 µg. Pregnancy 600 µg, lactation 500 µg.

Introduction

Table 3 *continued*

	Dietary sources	Main functions and effects of deficiency	UK adult RNI	USA adult RDA
Pantothenic acid	Widely distributed. Rich sources: yeast, offal, peanuts, meat, eggs, green vegetables.	Co-enzyme in energy metabolism. *Deficiency:* no specific deficiency identified.	No RNI. 3–7 mg assumed adequate.	5 mg. Pregnancy 6 mg, lactation 7 mg.
C (ascorbic acid)	Fruit, fruit juice, and vegetables, including potatoes.	Structure and maintenance of blood vessels, muscles, bone cartilage. Antioxidant and promotes absorption of non-haem iron. *Deficiency:* scurvy, poor wound healing, subcutaneous haemorrhage.	40 mg. Pregnancy 50 mg, lactation 70 mg.	75 mg. Pregnancy 85 mg, lactation 120 mg.

[a] $1 \mu g = 0.001$ mg.
[b] Chemical names are given in parentheses.
[c] PUFA, polyunsaturated fatty acids.

As the sciences of biochemistry and genetics have become more advanced, the case for supplementation to 'optimum' level has been put forward more strongly for certain vitamins such as vitamin C, folic acid, B_6, and possibly B_{12}. Vitamins A, C, and E have become known as the 'antioxidant' vitamins. These will be discussed in detail elsewhere in the book.

In high doses some vitamins can be toxic. This is most likely with fat-soluble vitamins, especially vitamin A, where high doses in early pregnancy can cause malformations in the fetus. Women are therefore advised not to eat liver in early pregnancy due to its high content of vitamin A. Cases of vitamin D toxicity are rare, but in the post-war years when the vitamin was added to baby foods and given as a supplement, cases of hypercalcaemia (due to the vitamin's effects on calcium absorption) were seen. Water-soluble vitamins are less likely to cause problems because they are not generally stored in the body, but very high doses of vitamin C (over 2 g per day) will cause gastrointestinal upsets, and it has been suggested that vitamin B_6 taken in very high doses to prevent menstrual symptoms in women may have ill-effects on the nervous system.

More information about specific vitamin and mineral supplements is given elsewhere (see p. 162).

NON-NUTRIENT SUBSTANCES IN FOODS

There are a whole range of biologically active substances in foods, especially plant foods and herbal remedies, apart from those accepted as nutrients. Some of these are harmful or affect the availability of nutrients in the diet, but others may have beneficial effects on health. Many of the active substances have been isolated and are now available as dietary supplements; however, their presence, previously unrecognized, is probably the best advertisement there is for eating a varied diet, including plenty of vegetables, pulses, and fruits, as it is quite possible that there are still other substances that remain to be discovered. Much of the evidence for the benefit of such substances has come from epidemiological studies, where the prevalence of certain types of disease is related to the consumption of specific foods or food groups within the community. Further scientific study is then needed to identify the particular active component and demonstrate an effect in the body. The following paragraphs outline the importance of some of the compounds that have been studied more extensively.

Antioxidants

Oxidation is an essential process whereby the nutrients we obtain from foods are oxidized in a controlled manner involving the consumption of oxygen. Carried out at a cellular level, oxidation releases energy for metabolism and transformation of nutrients into body tissue and generation of heat. The oxygen is ultimately converted into water and excreted. However, during this process so-called free radicals or reactive oxygen species are formed that, unless mopped up by the body's antioxidant defences, can damage the tissues, increasing the rate at which they age and potentially contributing to a range of degenerative diseases such as arthritis, immune disorders, cancer, stroke, coronary heart disease, and many others. Antioxidants are substances pro-

Introduction

duced by the body, or consumed in foods, that significantly delay or prevent the oxidation of a particular substrate.

Some vitamins and trace elements in the diet contribute to the body's antioxidant arsenal. Vitamins A (as beta-carotene), C, and E are known as the antioxidant vitamins, and selenium, copper, manganese, and zinc are components of antioxidant enzymes. In fact the carotenoids, the red–orange pigments in plants, comprise about 600 different substances, of which about 60 are precursors of vitamin A. Many of the non-provitamin carotenoids, including substances such as lycopene, zeaxanthin, and lutein act as antioxidants. Lycopene is the most interesting of these. It is present in tomatoes and, therefore, in food products such as ketchup and sauces. Cooking releases the lycopene and makes it more available, especially in the presence of a small amount of oil or fat. Recent epidemiological studies have suggested that consumption of tomatoes and products containing them is associated with a lower incidence of prostate cancer. Consumption of 10 or more servings per week of foods containing tomatoes, including soup, pizza, and pasta sauces afforded the greatest protection. In addition, non-nutrients such as phytoestrogens, flavonoids, phenolic acids, and polyphenols such as tannins are present in foods and drinks, and may help to prevent oxidation in the plant as well as in human tissues.

Flavonoids

Flavonoids are phenolic compounds that are water soluble and occur widely in nature. There are hundreds of different flavonoids found in fruits, vegetables, and beverages such as tea and wine. The particular flavonoids in tea and wine have strong antioxidant effects. Epidemiological studies have suggested that the risk of coronary heart disease is substantially lower in people within populations with the highest flavonoid intake, possibly due to the prevention of oxidation of low-density lipoproteins and reducing blood clotting. The most widely distributed flavonoid in foods is quercitin, followed by kaempferol, but others include myrecitin, catechin, apeginin, and luteolin. In a Dutch study investigating flavonoid intakes, black tea was found to supply more than half the intake, followed by onions and apples (see also p. xxxi).

Phytoestrogens

Phytoestrogens are steroid substances derived from plants, that, it has been suggested, have several potentially beneficial actions in the body. Epidemiological studies suggest that in populations where there is a high intake of phytoestrogens the incidence of certain cancers, especially hormone-sensitive types such as some forms of breast cancer and ovarian cancer in women and prostate cancer in men, is lower. One group, known as lignans, are derived from the bacterial digestion of polyphenols, and many oilseeds such as soya bean, rapeseed, and flax are rich sources of the lignans or their precursors. Women in countries with high consumption of soya beans and soya products have been shown to have a lower incidence of breast cancer. This may be related to the phytoestrogen content of the foods as well as to the presence of flavonoids and other phenolic compounds. Soya is also a rich source of another class of phytoestrogens – the isoflavonoids – especially diadzein and genistein.

Phytoestrogens appear to increase the binding of sex hormones to the protein on which they are carried in the blood, thus resulting in lower levels of biologically active free hormone, but they also have other potentially beneficial effects. Some have antioxidant effects that are cancer-preventing, while others appear to reduce the proliferation of cells that respond to oestrogens (such as in the breast and uterus) either by inhibiting enzymes involved in cell proliferation or by competing with oestrogens for binding sites. Food manufacturers are taking the opportunity to make products in which the above potentially beneficial components of foods are concentrated naturally, or are adding them to other foods. For example, soya, flax, and linseed may be added to breads to increase the phytoestrogen content, with the breads then being advertised as functional foods.

Phytoestrogens are also regarded as active principles in herbal remedies (see p. xxxii).

FUNCTIONAL FOODS

These are foods that appear to have health benefits beyond the provision of nutrients and energy. A recent symposium on the topic gave the following definition 'a food can be said to be functional if it contains a compound, which may or may not be a nutrient, that affects one or a limited number of functions in the body in a targeted way so as to have positive effects on health'. The health benefits may be physiological or may take the form of a positive psychological effect.

Functional foods may be foods that contain the beneficial substance naturally, e.g. fruits and vegetables contain a variety of antioxidant substances that are not strictly nutrients but have beneficial effects: wholegrain cereals contain dietary fibre that may have beneficial effects on gut function and help prevent heart disease; soya beans contain phytoestrogens that may have beneficial effects as described above. However, increasingly food manufacturers are producing foodstuffs with 'functional' added ingredients that may be of benefit to health. For example, spreads with plant sterols or plant stanols added may help lower

Introduction

cholesterol levels; addition of specific bacteria, called probiotics, to yoghurts and yoghurt drinks, may have beneficial effects within the gut and beyond; and chewing gum containing phosphatidylcholine is claimed to improve memory.

Legislative bodies in most countries are currently struggling to define the health claims that may be made for such foods, and to describe the evidence that is needed before such claims can be made. In the UK a voluntary code, 'The Joint Health Claims Initiative', has been developed by manufacturers working with the scientific community and consumer groups, which describes the types of claims, that can be made. In the USA the Food and Drugs Administration adjudicates on claims, and in other countries specific bodies have also been set up to advise on the subject.

In this book functional foods are discussed where appropriate – whether as foods such as cholesterol-lowering spreads, fish oils, cereals, probiotic yoghurts, and many others, or as products containing herbal materials, such as drinks containing ginkgo or echinacea, which may also put them into the category of functional food.

DIETARY RECOMMENDATIONS

Dietary recommendations come in various forms. Most countries produce specific guidelines for energy and nutri-ent intake for men and women and different age groups. These are usually referred to as recommended daily amounts, but are expressed differently in different countries. For example, in the USA RDAs for the average amount of energy required for a particular group are given, together with recommendations for nutrient intakes sufficient to cover the needs of those people in each group with the highest requirements. In the UK, since 1991, a slightly different approach has been taken in order to take account of variation in nutrient requirements between individuals. Here three different sets of nutrient requirements are given with the highest, the reference nutrient intake, corresponding to the recommended daily allowances. It is important to remember that these guidelines are for populations, not individuals – they cannot take into account individual factors such as size and exercise patterns.

Other types of recommendations outline the composition of diets that might be expected to prevent diseases such as coronary heart disease, obesity, and hypertension. Public health organizations in the UK, USA, and internationally have produced such guidelines. The World Health Organization Guidelines from 1990 are shown in Table 4; others may differ slightly in detail but are broadly similar.

Often, for general education purposes, these guidelines are translated into food groups, indicating which foods

Table 4 Nutrient intake goals

	Limits of population average intakes[a]	
	Lower	Upper
Total fat (% of total energy)[b]	15	30[c]
Saturated fatty acids (% of total energy)	0	10
Polyunsaturated fatty acids (% of total energy)	3	7
Dietary cholesterol (mg per day)	0	300
Total carbohydrate (% of total energy)	55	75
Complex carbohydrate[d] (% of total energy)	50	70
Free sugars (% of total energy)	0	10
Dietary fibre		
as total dietary fibre (g per day)	27	40
as non-starch polysaccharides (g per day)	16	24
Proteins (% of total energy)	10	15
Salt (g per day)	–	6

[a] Desirable lower and upper limits.

[b] Assumes sufficient energy is supplied for normal childhood growth, the needs of pregnancy and lactation, for work and desirable physical activities, and to maintain appropriate body reserves.

[c] Interim goal for countries with high fat intakes; further benefits expected by reducing intake towards 15% of total energy.

[d] The diet should include a daily minimum of 400 g of fruits and vegetables, of which at least 30 g should be pulses, nuts, and seeds.

Source: World Health Organization (1990). *Diet, nutrition and the prevention of chronic diseases*. WHO technical report, no. 797. WHO, Geneva.

Introduction

should be the major component of the diet and those that should ideally be used in smaller amounts because they contain large quantities of fat and sugar. These guidelines attempt to indicate the types of foods that would result in a healthy diet, rather than simply covering the requirements for energy and nutrients. Such guidelines are often produced in pictorial form – in the UK a plate model called 'The balance of good health' is used, with large slices for foods such as vegetables and fruit and starchy foods, smaller slices for meat, fish, and dairy foods, and fine slivers for fats and sugar. In the USA a food pyramid is preferred, with the starchy foods and fruit and vegetables at the base, and oil, fats, and sugars at the top.

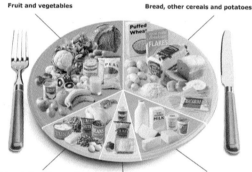

The Balance of Good Health

Fruit and vegetables

Bread, other cereals and potatoes

Meat, fish and alternatives

Foods containing fat
Foods and drinks containing sugar

Milk and dairy foods

There are five main groups of valuable foods

The USA Food Pyramid

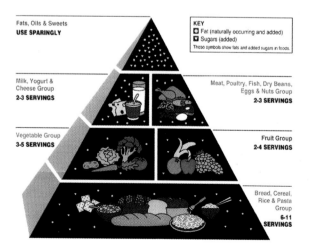

READING THE LABELS

Food labels often include information about both the ingredients and the nutritional content. There are regulations concerning the use of these, which in the UK are encompassed in the Food Labelling Regulations 1996.

Ingredients' lists inform the consumer about the foods that are present in a composite food or dish. They are listed in order of weight, the first item being present in the greatest amount and the last in the smallest amount. Food additives that are used in the formulation of the product must also be listed. However, this does not mean that you can assume that if an additive is not listed it will not be present. This is because if an ingredient that is used in the food already has an additive in it, the latter need not be listed. For example, if self-raising flour was an ingredient, the new ingredient list would simply list flour, but not the raising agent in the self-raising flour. This could be important if a person was intolerant to small amounts of the unlisted ingredient.

Nutrition labelling has been a contentious issue for years, There is evidence to suggest that people find the nutrition information difficult to understand. The UK regulations state that if nutritional labelling is to be used it must include the energy and the main nutrients supplying the energy, i.e. protein, fat, and carbohydrate. This information must be given as energy (in kcal and kJ) and nutrients per 100 g of food. Manufacturers can add other information if they so wish. Thus a typical label might read as in Table 5.

The difficulty here is that many people find it confusing to work out how much of the energy and nutrients are present in the portion that they are eating – for example, how many grams does a slice of ham or a bowl of cereal weigh? Some manufacturers will therefore add extra information; e.g. for a breakfast cereal the information may be given for a portion as well as the required value (see Table 6).

Table 5 Nutrition information (per 100 g of food)

Energy	665 kJ, 157 kcal
Protein	6.3 g
Fat	3.1 g
of which saturates	1.6 g
monounsaturates	0.5 g
polyunsaturates	1.0 g
Carbohydrate	25.8 g
of which sugars	9.5 g
starch	16.3 g
Fibre (as non-starch polysaccharide)	3.9 g

Red is essential, green is voluntary.

Introduction

Information about the content of vitamins and minerals is not essential but if given this must also show the proportion of the recommended daily allowance (where there is one) that 100 g of food supplies (see Tables 7 and 8).

There are a range of other regulations that govern potentially misleading claims (e.g. 'low fat', 'no added sugar or salt', 'increased fibre') that manufacturers wish to put on their labels or use in advertising. In one particular case manufacturers claimed that a food was x% fat-free. A food that claims to be, e.g., '92% fat-free' sounds good, but it still contains 8 g of fat per 100 g of food, which is a substantial amount of fat and energy. '% fat-free' claims are no longer allowed. Table 9 shows the current UK requirements.

Table 6 Nutrition information: for a serving (30 g) of Fibrepops[a] plus 125 ml of semi-skimmed milk

Energy	613 kJ, 144 kcal
Protein	7.8 g
Fat	2.8 g
of which saturates	1.4 g
monounsaturates	0.7 g
polyunsaturates	0.4 g
Carbohydrate	23.6 g
of which sugars	11.9 g
starch	11.7 g
Fibre (as non-starch polysaccharide)	5.6 g[b]

[a] A fictitious cereal.
[b] In the USA fibre is given as total dietary fibre (see p. xv)

Table 7 Nutrient content (per 100 g of food)

Sodium	0.6 g	
Vitamin D	4.3 µg	(85% RDA)
Thiamin (B$_1$)	1.2 mg	(85% RDA)
Folic acid	200 µg	(100% RDA)
Iron	11.9 mg	(85% RDA)

Table 8 Nutrition information: for a serving (30 g) of Fibrepops plus 125 ml of semi-skimmed milk

Sodium	0.2 g	
Vitamin D	0.6 µg	(12% RDA)
Thiamin (B$_1$)	0.3 mg	(21% RDA)
Folic acid	75 µg	(38% RDA)
Iron	4.9 mg	(35% RDA)

Table 9 Explanations of some label claims[a]

	Low	No added	Free from[b]
Fat	No more than 3 g fat per 100 g or 100 ml	–	No more than 0.15 g per 100 g or 100 ml
Sugars	No more than 5 g per 100 g or 100 ml	No sugars, or foods containing mainly sugars, added to the food or its ingredients	No more than 0.2 g per 100 g or 100 ml
Salt/sodium	No more than 40 mg sodium per 100 g or 100 ml	No sodium or salt added to the food or its ingredients	No more than 5 mg sodium per 100 g or 100 ml

Fibre

To claim	'Source of fibre'	'Increased fibre'	'High fibre'
	3 g per 100 g or 100 ml, or at least 3 g in the reasonable expected daily intake of the food	At least 25% more than a similar food for which no claim is made, and at least 3 g in the reasonable daily intake of the food if this is less than 100 g or 100 ml	Either at least 6 g per 100 g or 100 ml or at least 6 g in the reasonable daily intake of the food

[a] UK Food Labelling Standards, 1999.
[b] Levels allowed if the food is claimed to be 'free from' the particular nutrient.

Introduction

Herbal medicine

A short history of medicine

Doctor, I have an earache.

2000 BC Hear, eat this root.

AD 1000 That root is heathen. Hear, say this prayer.

AD 1850 That prayer is superstition. Hear, drink this potion.

AD 1940 That potion is snake oil. Hear, swallow this pill.

AD 1985 That pill is ineffective. Hear, take this antibiotic.

AD 2000 That antibiotic is artificial. Hear, eat this root.

Author unknown

As with food, the earliest human beings collected plants to be used as medicine. Although it is not clear why certain species were chosen, no doubt trial and error played an important part. At the beginning, and still today, plants for herbal medicine were and may be collected locally; however, the development of trade and migrations between countries and continents has led to a utilization of foreign material.

Some of the earliest writings on medicinal plants were produced in China, Egypt, and India hundreds of years BC. In the first century AD, the Greek physician Dioscorides wrote the first European herbal, listing about 600 herbs. This work influenced Western medicine for a very long time.

In the nineteenth century conventional medicine started to outstrip herbalism, at least in Western culture. Nevertheless, in Europe, North America, and some other countries there is still a strong interest in plant medicines – indeed, there is an increasing appreciation, because of a desire on the part of consumers to return to a more natural life-style and because, rightly or wrongly, modern synthetic medicines are often considered too expensive, and give rise to unwanted side-effects. In some parts of the world (e.g. India, China, Africa) herbalism still overshadows conventional medicine; about 80% of the population of developing countries depend on herbal medicine. The laws concerning the practice of herbal medicine vary according to the country – in some the practice must be carried out by qualified physicians. World-wide, the trade in herbal medicines runs into billions of dollars.

The herbal medicine practitioner will start with the plant or parts of the plant (seeds, roots, etc.) and then prepare the herbal medicine. For this activity to be successful,

certain precautions are necessary. Exact identification of the material is required.

The vast majority of medicinal plants are angiosperms (flowering plants), and are classified into family/genus/species. A well-known herb is Roman chamomile. This belongs to the family Compositae (term normally used in Europe)/Asteraceae (term normally used in North America). Some other families, too, have alternative names, which, if they exist, are also used in this book. The genus of Roman chamomile is *Chamaemelum*, the species is *nobile*. This is the so-called 'binomial nomenclature'. Latin, rather than common names are given to enable communication at an international level. In some cases alternative Latin names – called synonyms – have been used commonly for herbs. Botanists recognize a preferred or correct name for a plant, on the basis of first publication and other criteria.

In the present book the description of the example given would be:

Roman chamomile
Chamaemelum nobile syn. *Anthemis nobilis*
Family Compositae/Asteraceae

As far as the herbs in this book are concerned, only commonly encountered synonyms are given.

Clearly, for efficient quality control medicinal plants and their products must be identified and labelled correctly, preferably with the Latin name. The identification of the members of some families (e.g. Umbelliferae/Apiaceae; Compositae/Asteraceae) does require good botanical knowledge; consequently, physicians in past times received training in botany. A complete medicinal plant may be identified on external features, but plant parts, powdered material, and other products (tablets, capsules, tinctures, etc.) can usually only be identified using microscopy and chemical analysis (usually a form of chromatography). Adulteration can be a problem, particularly when the adulterant is of a toxic nature; e.g. burdock root adulterated with deadly nightshade root. One presumes that a reputable supplier of herbal products carries out a comprehensive quality control. Other conditions that can affect the chemical constituents of a herbal preparation include the environment in which the plant was growing, and there can also be variation between the members of a species.

Many medicinal plants are still collected in the wild, although there is also cultivation of some, of which a very

Introduction

good example is ginkgo. One interesting project, being carried out with the co-operation of the Royal Botanic Gardens at Kew, is the Living Pharmacy in the city of Fortaleza, and other cities, in north-east Brazil. In the Living Pharmacy, medicinal plants, both native and foreign, are cultivated in botanic gardens. These provide medicines for local people unable to meet the cost of conventional medicines. In many countries where the harvesting of wild plants takes place, there is worry about conservation and, as a result, some regulations have come into force.

Medicinal herbs were used for centuries without people knowing the reasons for their activity. It was at about the beginning of the nineteenth century that chemical investigations led to the identification of constituents, some of which were supposed to be 'active principles' – chemical constituents that have a healing or therapeutic effect. Plants contain thousands of chemical substances, and the claims that some are active principles have not always been supported by scientific investigation.

Because of improving methods of analysis, many types of substances have been identified in plants. As stated earlier, the present book is meant for the general reader, and therefore a simplified list of presumed active principles is presented below.

1. *Alkaloids*. These include some of the first active principles isolated from plants, e.g. morphine from opium (about 1800). They contain nitrogen. Plants that possess alkaloids tend to be toxic but, nevertheless, some are used in herbal medicine and are available, e.g. lobelia, comfrey, and borage. Some alkaloids can affect the liver; consequently, herbal products containing these substances should be treated with great caution, and indeed are by professional herbalists.

2. *Phenols*. A number of different types of phenolic substances are regarded as active principles.
   (a) Simple phenols: e.g. salicylic acid in willow – the forerunner of aspirin.
   (b) Tannins: very widespread in herbal plants and used commercially to convert hides into leather. Tannins are 'astringent', i.e. they harden and tighten skin and internal delicate (mucous) membranes. They are claimed to be antiseptic, to reduce bleeding, and to control diarrhoea. Tannins are said to function as antioxidants. The 'French paradox' refers to the lower than expected rate of heart disease in France, despite a relatively high-fat diet. This has been correlated with the high consumption of red wine, which is rich in tannins. Grapeseed products, also rich in tannins, have been developed in France as a health food.
   (c) Coumarins: responsible for the smell of new-mown hay. Scopoletin, found in cramp bark and black haw, shows antispasmodic (controls spasms and cramps) activity; it has also been claimed, from animal studies, that this particular coumarin exhibits anti-inflammatory and analgesic (pain-reducing) properties. Dicoumarol, formed from coumarin in spoiled sweet clover hay, is a potent blood anti-clotting drug and its discovery led to the development of modern anticoagulants.
   (d) Anthraquinones: active principles in well known laxative drugs, e.g. cascara, senna, and aloe.
   (e) Flavonoids: very widely distributed in plants, and some constitute the white, yellow, red, purple, and blue flower and fruit pigments. Numerous properties have been attributed to flavonoids, such as being antibacterial, anticancer, antiviral, anti-inflammatory, and that they bring about a reduction in blood capillary fragility, thus improving microcirculation. Flavonoids are claimed to be antioxidants.

3. *Essential (volatile) oils and resins.*
   (a) Essential oils contain terpenoids (monoterpenes and sesquiterpenes). In food, they are well known flavourings, e.g. cinnamon, clove, and mint. As regards herbal medicine: some (e.g. fennel and peppermint) are used as carminatives (they relieve digestive gas or wind and indigestion); some stimulate the gastric juices (e.g. sweet flag); and others (e.g. chamomile) are said to be antispasmodic and anti-inflammatory. The essential oil produced by mustard is used as a rubefacient (it brings blood to the skin and causes reddening and warming) and a counter-irritant (irritant to the skin, supposed to relieve deep-seated problem). Garlic essential oil has many herbal uses.

      Steam distillation is employed to isolate essential oils from the plant, and consequently great care must be taken with some 'neat' oils: e.g. thujone in wormwood and sage oil (notorious in the liqueur absinthe), while safrole in sassafras oil is carcinogenic.
   (b) Resins: sticky, solid substances, and a mixture of chemicals. A well known example is propolis (bee glue).

4. *Saponins and cardioactive chemicals.*
   (a) Saponins produce frothing in water. Steroidal saponins (e.g. in yam) can be used to make sex and other hormones.

Introduction

(b) Cardioactive drugs are steroids that strengthen a weakened heart. Digoxin is extracted from a foxglove species (*Digitalis lanata*) but, because of the powerful action and legal restrictions, herbalists are very cautious about using *Digitalis*. Hawthorn is a cardioactive herbal.

5. *Cyanogenetic glycosides, iridoids, and bitter principles.*
   (a) A cyanogenetic glycoside yields toxic prussic acid on hydrolysis. Cassava is a well known food plant that contains a cyanogenetic glycoside, but processing removes the prussic acid. Apricot seed kernels possess amygdalin, a cyanogenetic glycoside, once claimed as a treatment for cancer but now disproved.
   (b) Iridoids are said to be the active principles of valerian and devil's claw, and possess sedative properties.
   (c) Bitter principles are a range of chemical compounds. Plants containing (e.g. bitter quassia) are used for their appetite-stimulating properties, which may lead to better health.

6. *Mucilage.* Mucilage contains carbohydrates, and in herbal medicine is used for its demulcent (soothing) action on inflamed conditions of the digestive tract. It can also function as a laxative. Marshmallow and ispaghula are examples of mucilage-containing plants.

7. *Phytoestrogens.* These affect reproductive and sex hormone activity. Examples are the isoflavonoids found in soya and red clover, which may have potential as cancer-treating chemicals.

8. *Inorganic elements.* Plants possess a very wide range of inorganic elements, some of which are claimed to play an important part in herbal medicine; e.g. iodine in seaweeds.

In health food stores, pharmacies, and supermarkets herbal products are usually available as extracts (e.g. tablets, capsules, teas, tinctures, lotions, ointments, lozenges, syrups). Many of these are sold without prescription as over-the-counter products. The legal situation regarding these products varies according to the country. In the USA most herbal extracts are sold as dietary supplements, which are a food category. Labelling may only refer to the effects on the structure or function of the body – therapeutic claims are not allowed. Herbal medicines in the UK fall into two categories: (a) licensed products that are required to meet safety, quality, and efficacy criteria, in a similar manner to any other licensed medicines; (b) the majority of herbal products, which are not licensed and are therefore sold as dietary supplements with no thera-peutic claims on the label; however, somewhat devious methods of advertising have been employed. In Germany and some other European Union countries, herbal medicinal products are treated in the same way as any other medicinal products and must satisfy, as a pre-condition for marketing, the same criteria of safety, quality, and efficacy as any other medicine. Efforts are being made to harmonize the situation within the European Union but this will probably take a long time.

The development of a new medical drug by a pharmaceutical company is a long and expensive process, taking between 10 and 12 years and costing about £350 million (US$600 million). It involves a survey of a large number of potentially useful chemicals, and animal and human (clinical) trials, before a licence can be granted by bodies such as the US Food and Drug Administration, or the UK Medicines Control Agency. Similar bodies exist in other countries. The development of a herbal product does not usually seem to appeal to major pharmaceutical companies, because of the cost involved, the complexity of the chemical make-up of the product, and the difficulty of patenting. Nevertheless, the marketing of herbal medicines is now attracting the attention of some large pharmaceutical companies.

In those countries where herbal medicines may be licensed, proof of efficacy (ability to achieve claimed actions) can be obtained from experiments and clinical studies (animal and human), and if these are not fully available then consideration is given to traditional experience of the product.

Germany has a long history of using herbal medicines. In the late 1970s an expert committee of physicians, pharmacists, and others was established to report on the safety and efficacy of a number of herbal medicines. The results were published as the Commission E monographs, later translated into English in the USA. These monographs were comprehensive, covering uses, contraindications (interference with existing conditions), side-effects, interactions with other drugs, chemical constituents, and dosage. The information was taken from clinical studies and other sources. Monographs were produced on about 400 herbal medicines, about a third of which were not approved. Another similar project is the European Scientific Cooperative on Phytotherapy (ESCOP) which, in addition to other activities, has produced a number of herbal monographs.

Even if herbal products are sold as dietary supplements, i.e. without therapeutic claims, there is usually information on dosage, often with a statement of standardization to the presumed active principles. Clearly,

Introduction

dosage is important for all medicines, and for herbals it is one area that could warrant further research. A number of the German Commission E monographs refer to different ginkgo extracts, but only one is supported. Some herbal products are mixtures of species, and it is difficult in these cases to be clear about the active principles involved. When presumed active principles have been isolated from herbal material, they do not necessarily have the same therapeutic effect as the complete material, which suggests that either the presumption is wrong or that the therapeutic effect is the result of an interaction between the chemical substances in a herb.

In Western countries, physicians vary in their interest in herbal medicine. Some 70% of physicians in Germany prescribe herbal products; in the UK there is an increasing but still limited interest. Whatever the situation, a patient should tell his or her doctor if herbal medicines are being used, because they may interact with the synthetic medicine being prescribed. This, of course, assumes that the physician has a knowledge of herbal medicines. It must be realized that a patient may feel that a herbal medicine is producing good results. This could well be a psychological (a placebo) rather than a physiological effect; nevertheless, in some situations this might be a satisfactory state of affairs.

The published literature reveals a vast number of scientific and clinical investigations into herbal products, although these may be restricted with certain species. There seems to be a place for herbal medicine in our culture, but more research is required into certain aspects, such as active principles, purification, dosage, and control. It should be pointed out that self-diagnosis and self-medication can be dangerous – a number of fatalities have occurred through the ingestion of herbal products, and many herbal medicines should not be taken during pregnancy and lactation (breastfeeding). Expert advice should always be sought. In some countries, e.g. Germany, a physician may have had training in herbal medicine; in others this may not be the case, and in those situations an approach should be made to an experienced and professional herbalist. For example, in the UK there is the National Institute of Medical Herbalists, whose members observe a strict code of ethics.

In the present book, some 100 herbal medicines (presently available) are described, covering a range of situations. As far as possible, the scientific evidence for the claimed efficacy is given. The Recomended reading section (see p. 173) provides information on many more herbal preparations, dosages, side-effects, contraindications, and interactions.

Alfalfa, lucerne *Medicago sativa*

Family Leguminosae/Fabaceae

ORIGIN AND CULTIVATION

Alfalfa does not exist in the truly wild state. It is said to have originated in the area around the Caspian Sea, possibly from the local *Medicago coerulea*. The cultivation and spread of alfalfa seems linked with the spread of the horse. The plant was taken to China from central Asia over 2000 years ago. Introduced to Greece from Persia in the fifth century BC, and then throughout Europe, it is now cultivated all over the world, mainly as an animal forage.

PLANT DESCRIPTION

Alfalfa is a perennial herb with a deep taproot and clover-like leaves (trifoliate), and grows to a height of 1 m (3 ft). The flowers are usually bluish purple but, because of hybridization with other species, may be variegated, with some yellow colour. Its coiled fruits are the typical leguminous pods, containing numerous greenish brown seeds, each about 2 mm in diameter.

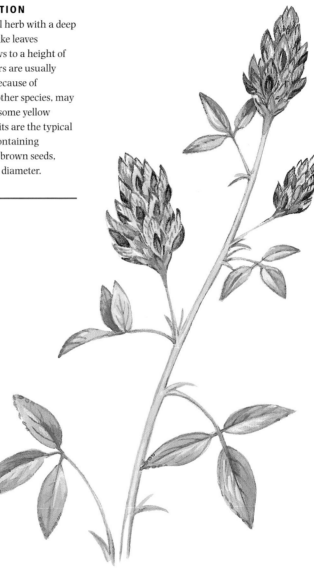

CULINARY AND NUTRITIONAL VALUE

Alfalfa is very important as a livestock forage. In some parts of the world the leaves are eaten raw or cooked as a vegetable in human diets. Seed sprouts are a favourite salad ingredient. Alfalfa extract is used as a flavouring agent in many food commodities, its leaf protein is used as a protein substitute in vegan diets, and its chlorophyll is employed as a colouring agent.

The plant has been subjected to numerous chemical analyses and has been shown to be rich in a variety of chemical substances; e.g. protein (14–15% in dried plant), minerals and trace elements, vitamins, saponins, flavonoids, coumarins, and numerous others. Sprouts contain a large amount of water (>90%), a small amount of protein (4%), and a range of minerals and vitamins (carotene, B, and C).

CLAIMS AND FOLKLORE

Alfalfa is available in the form of herbal teas, tablets, tinctures, and other preparations. Apart from its nutritional value, there are numerous anecdotal claims concerning its therapeutic usefulness. These relate to treatment of various arthritic conditions, skin ailments, and diabetes, to stimulating the appetite, to it being a general tonic, and to numerous other conditions.

EVIDENCE

There is really no scientific evidence to support the vast majority of therapeutic claims.

Animal experiments and a very few human experiments indicate that ingestion of alfalfa seeds may lower blood cholesterol, but more investigations are required. Those with a predisposition to systemic lupus erythematosus, and those who are photosensitive, should avoid alfalfa. Similarly, it is best avoided during pregnancy and lactation.

Algae

ORIGIN AND CULTIVATION

The algae constitute a large group of 'primitive' plants – they do not reproduce by seeds as in most medicinal and food plants but rather by spores, and the plant body is not divided into root, stem, and leaf, but is in the form of a relatively undifferentiated 'thallus'. They are mainly aquatic, being found in freshwater ponds, rivers, and lakes, and are the seaweeds found on shores all over the world.

Total seaweed usage alone amounts to about 3.5 million tons per year. In Western countries seaweeds are harvested from their natural habitats, but in Asia there is quite a good deal of planned cultivation (e.g. see *Porphyra* below). Although microscopic algae (*Chlorella* and *Spirulina*) may be harvested naturally, today they are usually cultivated commercially.

PLANT DESCRIPTION

Algae are classified according to their pigments. All algae contain the green pigment chlorophyll; the group known as the green algae contains only chlorophyll, but other groups have pigments in addition to chlorophyll. In the brown algae (seaweeds) the additional pigment is fucoxanthin. In the red algae (seaweeds) it is phycoerythrin (red) and phycocyanin (blue) – the relative quantities vary, so different species vary in colour from red to bluish green; in the blue-green algae the only extra pigment is phycocyanin. There is also great variation in size between species of the algae. Some are microscopic (unicellular and filamentous), whereas some seaweeds attain a length of 50 m (165 ft).

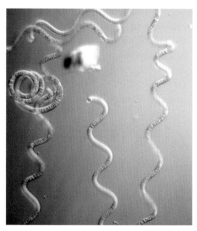

Spirulina, as seen with a microscope.

CULINARY AND NUTRITIONAL VALUE

Spirulina (a blue-green alga)

A microscopic, fresh-water alga found as corkscrew-like filaments. In the sixteenth century Spanish explorers found Aztecs harvesting a 'blue mud', probably consisting of *Spirulina*, from Lake Texaco (Mexico). This was dried and turned into chips and loaves. Similarly, the alga has been collected by local people from Lake Chad (Africa). *Spirulina* is still harvested from freshwater sources, but it is also cultured commercially in California, Thailand, India, and China. Presumably, it should be easier to produce a purer harvest from cultured material, rather than a natural source where other algae might be present.

The commercial product (the alga has been dried) contains: (a) 60–70% protein with a good amino acid profile; (b) 16–20% carbohydrate; (c) 2–3% fat; (d) 7–9% water; (e) 5–8% minerals, including iron, calcium, and many others; and (f) vitamins: beta-carotene (provitamin A) and some of the B complex, including, as reported, B_{12}, E, and K. The iron present is easily absorbed by humans, which is not always the case with iron from other plant sources. Vitamin B_{12} is not normally found in plant foods, only animal sources – a possible problem for vegetarians and vegans. However, as with *Chlorella* and seaweeds, there is considerable doubt about the nutritional significance of B_{12} recorded for *Spirulina*.

Spirulina presents a good nutritional profile, but it is far more expensive than some animal foods (e.g. meat, milk), which may not worry vegetarians.

Chlorella (a green alga)

A microscopic unicellular alga, up to about 10 μm (1 μm = 0.001 mm) in diameter. In many other respects it is similar to *Spirulina*. Commercial cultivation takes place, and its nutritional profile is roughly the same.

Both *Spirulina* and *Chlorella* are available as tablets in health food shops.

Seaweeds

The term 'kelp' is applied to a number of seaweed species. In many parts of the world seaweeds, often dried, are used directly in food – as vegetables, and in salads and soups. They are sometimes sold in health food shops, supermarkets, and similar establishments. The greatest usage is in the Orient; e.g. in Japan some 50 species are utilized.

Phycocolloids (carbohydrates) such as agars, alginates, and carrageenans are extracted from seaweeds and used as thickeners and stabilizers in a vast array of foods, including canned commodities, confectionery, ice-cream, jellies, soups, and sauces.

Generally speaking, seaweeds contain protein (amino acid profile similar to that of legumes), little fat, and some vitamins and minerals. Among the vitamins, B_{12} has been recorded but, as in *Spirulina*, its biological activity is open to debate. Of the minerals present, the relatively high concentration (0.07–0.76% dry weight) of iodine is of interest. Seaweeds in the diet provide fibre.

Below is information on some of the utilized seaweeds:

- Laver (*Porphyra umbilicalis*): a red seaweed, found on the rocky shores of the UK and other temperate North Atlantic countries. Its product is 'laver bread', particularly popular in south Wales but also eaten elsewhere.

Algae

- *Porphyra* is popular in China, Korea, and Japan (where it is known as *nori*). The Japanese cultivate *Porphyra* by sinking bundles of bamboo canes, brushwood, or nets offshore, to which will become attached a crop of the seaweed.

- Dulse (*Palmaria palmata* syn. *Rhodymenia palmata*): a red seaweed, consumed in the ways already described.

- Carrageen or Irish Moss (*Chondrus crispus*): a red seaweed collected commercially in Canada for carrageenan extraction. Small quantities are harvested in Ireland and France, and utilized as described on p. 2.

- Knotted wrack (*Ascophyllum nodosum*): a brown seaweed common in temperate Atlantic countries. It is harvested in Ireland, Scotland, and Norway for alginate extraction.

- Some other seaweed species utilized belong to *Laminaria* (in Japan known as *kombu*), *Macrocystis, Nereocystis, Fucus, Gelidium* (one source of agar), and *Undaria* (Jap. *wakame*).

Taking *Laminaria* (kelp) as an example of a seaweed, the nutrient analysis of fresh material is: water 81.6%; protein 1.7%; total fibre 1.33%; fat 0.6%; energy 43 kcal; 233 mg sodium; 168 mg calcium; 89 mg potassium; 2.9 mg iron; vitamin B_1 0.15 mg; vitamin B_2 0.47 mg; vitamin C 0.1 mg.

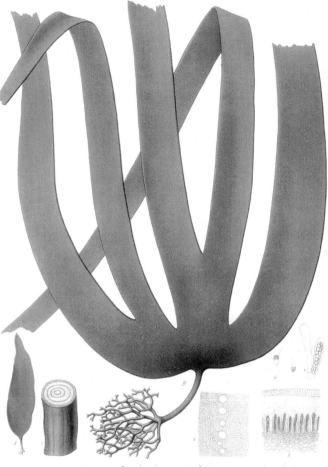

Laminaria, seaweed.

CLAIMS AND FOLKLORE

Spirulina, Chlorella, and kelp tablets are readily available. Kelp refers to a number of species, but usually to brown seaweeds. A considerable number of claims for the therapeutic value of *Spirulina* and *Chlorella* have been made, particularly on the Internet; one claim concerns the presence of vitamin B_{12}, normally found in animal tissues. Similarly, kelp products have been used to treat a large array of complaints, including obesity, rheumatism, arthritis, indigestion, constipation, and other problems. These treatments have often been related to the high concentration of iodine in seaweeds.

The phycocolloids (gels) present have a bulking effect in laxative preparations, and a demulcent action.

EVIDENCE

As stated earlier, the vitamin B_{12} reported for *Spirulina, Chlorella*, and seaweeds is not considered biologically active. The value of iodine as regards therapeutic claims for seaweed should be treated cautiously. Iodine is required by the thyroid gland to form the hormone thyroxine, which controls body metabolism. Deficiency leads to goitre, but in many countries this has been eliminated by fortification, such as by the use of iodized salt. However, deficiency of iodine can occur and kelp could provide the necessary iodine, but professional advice is required because too much iodine (above 150 µg per day) can lead to hyperthyroidism (weight loss, sweating, fatigue, and other symptoms). Iodine in kelp has somehow been related to the use of the product as a slimming aid in dealing with obesity. There seems little scientific support for this claim.

Seaweeds may absorb and concentrate unacceptable heavy metals, such as cadmium and lead, from contaminated sea water. Ingestion of kelp has been associated with the development of human acne.

Considering all the evidence, careful thought should go into the use of algal products. The therapeutic employment of kelp is not supported in Germany, and it should not be given during pregnancy and lactation.

Aloe   Aloe vera and other species

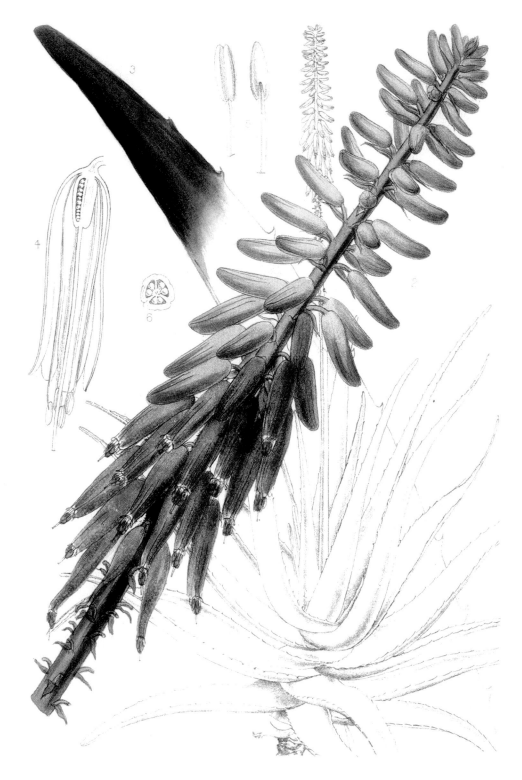

Aloe

Family Liliaceae

ORIGIN AND CULTIVATION

The *Aloe* species (about 300) are native to tropical and southern Africa, Madagascar, and Arabia, but have been introduced to many parts of the world. There are a number of ornamental species.

Two major products are derived from the leaves of *Aloe* species: (a) a yellow bitter juice from specialized cells beneath the leaf skin, or epidermis (this is processed to give the drug 'aloes', which is said to be obtained from all species); (b) a mucilaginous gel from the soft tissue in the centre of the leaf that gives the drug 'aloe vera' or 'aloe vera gel' (this is said to be, in the main, currently obtained from *Aloe vera* (Curaçao aloe or Barbados aloe) (syn. *A. barbadensis*), which is much cultivated in the New World tropics).

Other species of economic importance are *A. ferox* and its hybrids (Cape aloe, South Africa) and *A. perryi* (Socotrine or Zanzibar aloe).

PLANT DESCRIPTION

Aloe species are perennial succulents with dense rosettes of thick, spiky, grey green leaves with aerial stems bearing yellow, reddish, or orange tubular flowers. *A. vera* has 15–30 leaves, each up to 0.5 m ($1\frac{1}{2}$ ft) long and 8–10 cm (4 in) wide; the flowering stem is 60–90 cm (34 in) in height.

CULINARY AND NUTRITIONAL VALUE

The only culinary use of bitter 'aloes' (which must be highly diluted) is in beverages and confectionery to impart a bitter taste.

CLAIMS AND FOLKLORE

Aloe is of ancient usage. It has been identified in wall paintings of ancient Egypt dating to the fourth millennium BC. It was a traditional funeral gift for the pharaohs. In the Egyptian Book of Remedies (about 1500 BC), aloe was recommended for curing infections, treating skin disorders, and as a laxative. It was recorded in ancient Greece in the fourth century BC. The body of Jesus was wrapped in linen impregnated with myrrh and aloes. Dioscorides (about AD 74) used aloes to heal wounds, stop hair loss, treat genital ulcers, and eliminate haemorrhoids. In the sixth century Arab traders carried the plant to Asia and, in the sixteenth century, Spaniards transported it to the New World.

In more modern times, 'bitter aloes', which is obtained by allowing the yellow leaf juice to dry out and to give a brown mass, has been used as a purgative. Its action depends on the anthraquinones (glycosides) present.

'Aloe vera' gel (containing glucomannan and other polysaccharides, lipids, and some other substances) is used in the cosmetics industry in creams, shampoos, cleansers, soaps, and suntan lotions, with claims for moisturizing and revitalizing properties. It is claimed as a cure or remedy for burns, wounds, and various skin conditions (e.g. acne, dermatitis, psoriasis, hair loss).

Drinks containing 'aloe vera' are now available, and are said to relieve irritable bowel syndrome, peptic ulcers, and indigestion – and to be helpful for general detoxification!

EVIDENCE

There is no doubt that 'bitter aloes' is an effective laxative. Indeed, its purgative action is now usually considered too drastic, and other, milder laxatives are recommended. It should not be given to patients with haemorrhoids, or used during pregnancy and lactation.

A number of experimental investigations (both with animals and humans) have been carried out using 'aloe vera'. The results are difficult to interpret because (a) sometimes homogenized leaf extracts have been utilized, that contain both 'aloes' and 'aloe vera'; and (b) precise active constituents have not been isolated and characterized. In general, the literature on burn management and wound healing is confused, and further studies are required. However, the gel freshly extracted from the leaves is effective in dealing with minor burns – often as a home cure; it is hoped that 'aloe vera' in commercial preparations is stabilized and in sufficient concentration. There is a little support for 'aloe vera' gel as a remedy for acne and eczema.

Internal administration of 'aloe vera' (e.g. in drinks) does not seem to exert any consistent therapeutic effect.

External application of the gel during pregnancy and lactation would appear to be safe but internal administration, because of possible admixture with bitter 'aloes', is to be avoided.

Angelica Angelica archangelica;
dong quai A. sinensis syn. A. polymorpha var. sinensis

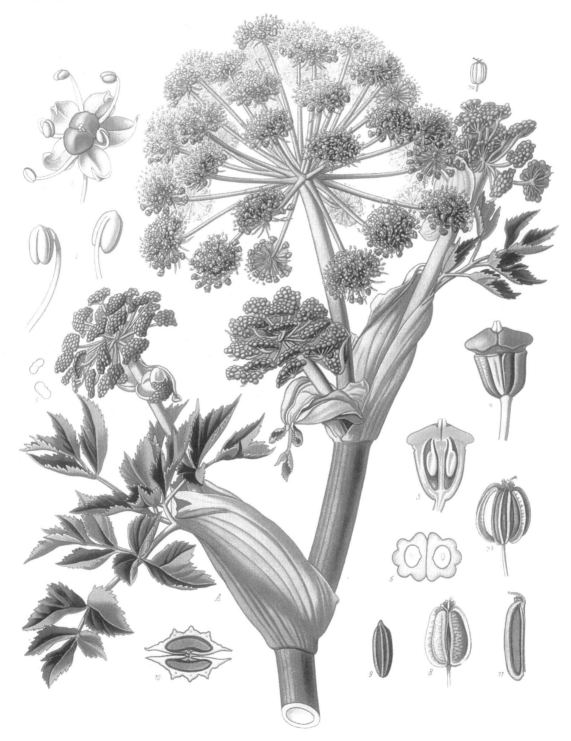

Angelica, dong quai

Family Umbelliferae/Apiaceae

ORIGIN AND CULTIVATION

- Angelica occurs wild in the colder parts of Europe, from Iceland, through Scandinavia, to central Russia; also in mountain ranges from the Pyrenees to Syria. It is found as an escapee from cultivation in many countries, including the UK. *A. atropurpurea* is utilized in the USA.

- Dong quai (*A. sinensis*) provides a popular drug in traditional Chinese medicine.

PLANT DESCRIPTION

- Angelica is a biennial growing to a height of 2 m ($6\frac{1}{2}$ ft) (when in flower). The green stems bear large bi- to tripinnate leaves that are 30–70 cm (28 in) long, and if the plant is allowed to grow into the second year, the flowering stems carry umbels of greenish white or green flowers, giving rise to 'seeds' (botanically speaking, these are fruits), 5–7 mm in length.

- Dong quai is a similar plant, with white flowers.

CULINARY AND NUTRITIONAL VALUE

Pieces of the young stem and leaf stalk of *A. archangelica* are candied (crystallized with sugar) and used in confectionery, their bright green colour being attractive. The roots may be used in making gin, and the 'seeds' vermouth and chartreuse.

CLAIMS AND FOLKLORE

- Angelica (*A. archangelica*): parts used are 'seed', leaf, rhizome, and root. It first became popular in Europe during the fifteenth century; it has been used internally for digestive disorders (e.g. gastric ulcers, anorexia), bronchitis, catarrh, flu, chronic fatigue, and menstrual and obstetric problems, and externally for rheumatic pain, neuralgia, and pleurisy.

- Dong quai (*A. sinensis*): the part used is the root. It is an important Chinese medical herb, its use dating back to about AD 200. It has been recommended for all kinds of gynaecological problems, and as an antispasmodic, a 'blood purifier', and for hypertension, rheumatism, and constipation.

EVIDENCE

Among the chemical substances present are coumarins and furancoumarins, and also a pleasant essential (volatile) oil. It is known that some coumarins can act as vasodilators and stimulate the central nervous system. However, the relatively few animal experiments carried out do not as yet justify all the claims for the efficacy of the herb.

The coumarins and furancoumarins, on contact with the skin, may lead to photosensitivity, which could result in a type of dermatitis that might become cancerous. This has given rise to a limit being recommended for root oil in cosmetic and suntan preparations.

Angelica products should not be used during pregnancy and lactation because of possible abortifacient effects. The root is recommended in Germany, for treatment of loss of appetite and flatulence, but not the 'seed' and overground parts.

Arnica, leopard's bane, mountain tobacco
Arnica montana, A. latifolia, A. sororia, A. fulgens, A. cordifolia

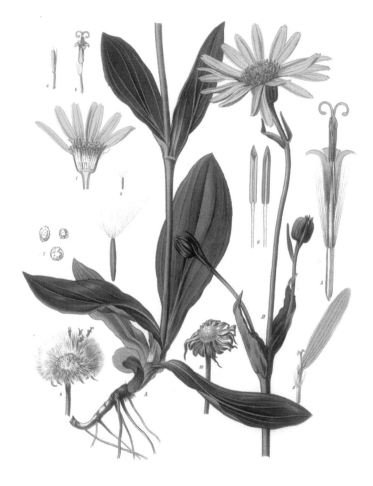

Family Compositae/Asteraceae

ORIGIN AND CULTIVATION
Arnica montana is found wild in mountainous regions of Europe; *A. latifolia*, *A. sororia*, *A. fulgens*, and *A. cordifolia* in western North America. Because of over-harvesting, collection of the plant is now subject to restriction in certain European countries. There is some experimental cultivation of arnica.

PLANT DESCRIPTION
Arnica is an herbaceous perennial with a basal rosette of ovate, hairy leaves 5–7 cm (3 in) in length, and growing to a height of 10–60 cm (24 in). The yellow flower heads are about 5 cm (2 in) across.

Herbal preparations are usually made from the flower heads, but also the roots and rhizomes.

CULINARY AND NUTRITIONAL VALUE
There is some use of the herb as a flavouring, but only in small quantities, and in alcoholic beverages.

CLAIMS AND FOLKLORE
At one time arnica was used for internal consumption, but this is no longer true because of its toxicity. An exception is its inclusion in homeopathic preparations, to be taken at the correct dilution. Its main function is to treat externally sprains, bruises, and unbroken chilblains, being included in ointments, salves, lotions, and tinctures.

EVIDENCE
Among the many chemical substances identified in arnica, the sesquiterpene lactones have been claimed to be the active principles. There is evidence from animal experiments that these are anti-inflammatory, analgesic, and antibacterial, which would support the external uses of arnica already described. However, in some cases arnica has caused allergic reactions. This may be important, because the herb has been included in some cosmetic preparations such as hair shampoos. It is approved in Germany.

It is worth restating that arnica should not be taken internally (except possibly in homeopathic preparations) because it is poisonous, leading to conditions such as shortage of breath, muscle paralysis (including the heart), and fatal gastroenteritis.

Artichoke (globe) *Cynara scolymus*

Family Compositae/Asteraceae

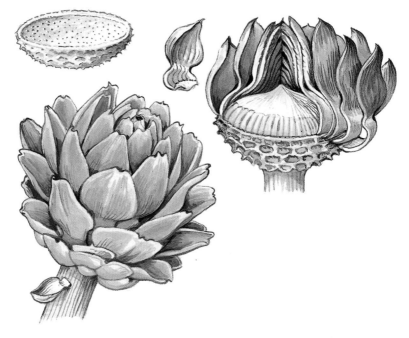

ORIGIN AND CULTIVATION
Cynara scolymus probably evolved in the Mediterranean region, maybe from a wild form of cardoon (*Cynara cardunculus*). The plant can be grown in many parts of Europe, but requires protection against frost. California is a major growing region. This artichoke should not be confused with Jerusalem artichoke (*Helianthus tuberosus*), also a member of the Compositae.

PLANT DESCRIPTION
It is an herbaceous perennial, 80–180 cm (70 in) in height, with greyish green, deeply lobed leaves, up to 75 cm (30 in) in length. The globose flower heads are 5–10 cm (4 in) in diameter, and consist of broad, fleshy, green scales or bracts surrounding the central violet–blue florets; both bracts and florets are attached to a receptacle or 'heart'.

CULINARY AND NUTRITIONAL VALUE
Artichoke was known as a food plant to the Greeks and Romans. The fleshy bases of the bracts and the receptacle are the parts usually eaten. They contain about 3% protein, 3% carbohydrate, little fat, and a small amount of vitamin C.

CLAIMS AND FOLKLORE
The plant parts used in herbal medicine are leaves, roots, and flower heads. Their extracts are said to be choleretic, i.e. they stimulate the liver and increase bile production; consequently, they have been used to treat chronic liver and gall bladder disease, jaundice, and some other conditions. They are also said to act as diuretics, and to reduce blood cholesterol and triglycerides.

EVIDENCE
Animal and human studies have supported some of the suggested functions of artichoke extracts, but there has also been conflicting evidence. The active principle is usually said to be cynarin (a phenolic acid), but other phenolic acids (chlorogenic and neochlorogenic) have also been implicated. In view of conflicting evidence, further research into the therapeutic value of artichoke is warranted. In Germany it is supported as a choleretic for dyspeptic problems. Excessive use of artichoke should be avoided during pregnancy and lactation.

Astragalus, milk vetch, huang qi

Astragalus membranaceus syn. A. propinguus; A. mongholicus syn.
A. membranaceus var. mongholicus; A. gummifer

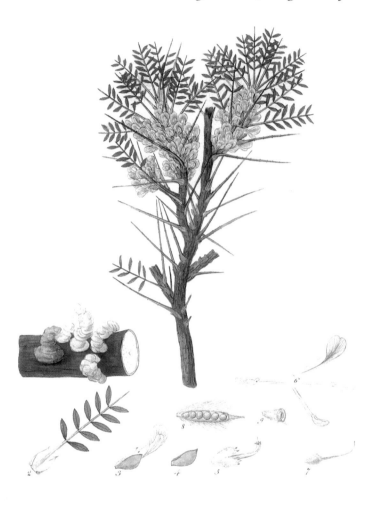

Family Leguminosae/Fabaceae

ORIGIN AND CULTIVATION

Some Chinese species, *Astragalus membranaceus*, *A. mongholicus*, and others, are native to northern China, and some to high regions such as Sichuan, Yunnan, and Tibet. *A. membranaceus* and *A. mongholicus* yield most of the root of commerce and are extensively cultivated. *A. gummifer* is found in the Middle East, particularly Kurdistan.

PLANT DESCRIPTION

A. membranaceus is a perennial growing to a height of about 40 cm (16 in), with grooved hairy stems and leaves divided into 12–18 pairs of leaflets. The yellow flowers are about 2 cm (1 in) long, giving rise to pendulous pods up to 15 cm (6 in) in length. The root is the source of herbal medicine. *A. gummifer* is an evergreen or semi-evergreen shrub growing to a height of 30 cm (12 in), with spiny, stalked pinnate leaves and clusters of white flowers.

NUTRITIONAL AND CULINARY VALUE

Tragacanth gum is obtained by tapping the branches and taproot of *A. gummifer*. It is used extensively in foods and ice-cream as an emulsifying, thickening, and suspending agent.

CLAIMS AND FOLKLORE

Tragacanth gum has been employed as a demulcent in cough and cold preparations, and as a treatment for diarrhoea. Some plant gums (e.g. guar) have been claimed to reduce serum lipid, cholesterol, and glucose levels. This is not the case with tragacanth, although the gum is non-toxic.

The roots of *A. membranaceus* and *A. mongholicus* contain a variety of chemical substances, such as saponins, polysaccharides, flavonoids, and others. They have been used for thousands of years in China as a tonic, particularly for young people, increasing endurance and improving resistance to cold temperatures.

Numerous claims have been made for the herb, e.g. that it improves resistance (immune response), possibly related to the polysaccharide content, and that it has antibacterial, antiviral, anti-inflammatory, and cardiovascular effects.

Astragalus extracts have been included in skin care products and hair tonics because of their presumed properties as vasodilators and sources of nourishment.

EVIDENCE

There is some experimental evidence (animal and human) to support the health claims.

Balm *Melissa officinalis*

Family Labiatae/Lamiaceae

ORIGIN AND CULTIVATION
The plant is native to southern Europe, western Asia, and North Africa, having been cultivated for over 2000 years. It was originally grown as a bee plant. Cultivation is probably now on a small scale.

PLANT DESCRIPTION
Balm grows to a height of 30–80 cm (30 in). It is a perennial that is lemon-scented when crushed, and bears ovate, pointed, and toothed leaves. The two-lipped flowers, about 12 mm ($\frac{1}{2}$ in) in length, are yellow at first but often change to white or pink.

The parts used in herbal medicine are the whole plant, or the leaves, or the essential oil.

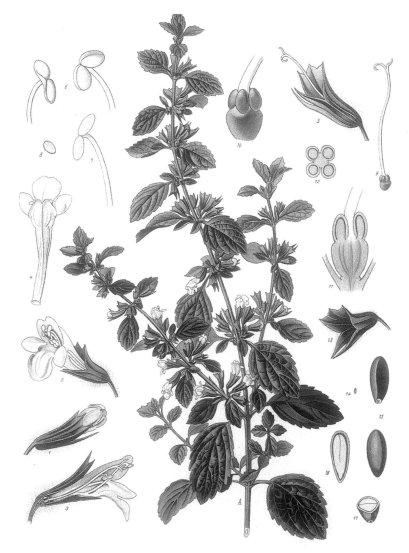

CULINARY AND NUTRITIONAL VALUE
The fresh leaves (lemon-scented) have been included in omelettes, salads, soups, sauces, herb vinegars, and game and fish dishes (especially in Spain), and in liqueurs such as Benedictine, Eau de Mélisse des Carmes, and Chartreuse.

CLAIMS AND FOLKLORE
Balm was well known to Arab physicians in the tenth and eleventh centuries.

The herb extract, has been taken internally, e.g. in herb tea, for nervous disorders, indigestion associated with such disorders, hyperthyroidism, depression, and anxiety; externally, the extract has been used for herpes, sores, and insect bites. In aromatherapy, the oil (up to 0.2% concentration) is used as a relaxant and to reduce nervous tension – it is said to be antispasmodic and antibacterial.

EVIDENCE
There is some experimental evidence that the herb extract is antiviral, which might explain its benefit regarding conditions such as herpes. Flavonoids and tannins have been implicated. In Germany, there is support for the use of the oil as a relaxant.

Bamboo *Bambusa arundinacea*

Family Gramineae/Poaceae

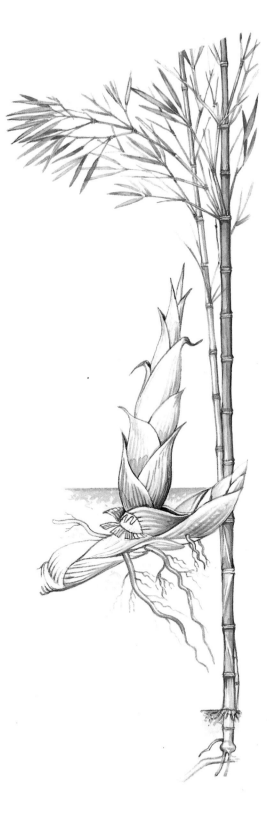

ORIGIN AND CULTIVATION
The bamboos are giant grasses, and there are about 500 species. They are found in China and Japan, and extending across Asia, and also in Africa and South America. Normally, bamboos grow in or near the tropics, but some of the hardier types can be cultivated in temperate regions.

PLANT DESCRIPTION
Some bamboos can grow to a height of 40 m (130 ft), with a daily growth of 40 cm (16 in). The stem is hollow and jointed, and there is a strong partition at each joint. Some bamboos flower every year; others, at intervals of 30 or 60 years.

The bamboo found in herbal medicine is described as *Bambusa arundinacea*.

CULINARY AND NUTRITIONAL VALUE
The young bamboo shoots are a popular food item in eastern Asia and in countries where Chinese cuisine is found. They are often canned. After harvesting, the shoots are boiled for about half an hour, to remove bitterness (cyanogenic glycosides) but to retain their crispness. The shoots contain about 3% protein, little fat, and about 5% carbohydrate, but only 4 mg per 100 g vitamin C. In some parts of the world, the seed (grain) has been used as food.

Bamboos have endless uses, e.g. building, baskets, ropes, and musical instruments.

CLAIMS AND FOLKLORE
In Ayurvedic (ancient Indian) medicine, the milky deposit or gum on the nodes of the stem was used as a cooling remedy for the lungs, and to treat a number of conditions, e.g. feverish colds and asthma. The claims made at present do not seem to be the same as in Ayurvedic medicine. Because it is rich in silica, it has been suggested that the gum can help bone and joint disorders, and that it may prevent bone loss after menopause.

EVIDENCE
There seems to be no experimental evidence to support the above claims.

Bee products

The use of honey bee products as food and medicine goes back thousands of years. In this account four items are considered: propolis, honey, pollen, and royal jelly. These items or their extracts are available commercially. As explained in the Introduction, they may be regarded as foods or dietary supplements rather than medicines, depending on the country.

Propolis (bee glue)

ORIGIN

Propolis is a brown, sticky, resinous substance collected by worker bees on their hind legs from the buds and barks of various trees – poplar (*Populus*) is a common source in temperate countries. In the hive, propolis is used to close cracks in the wall, sometimes to make the entrance smaller, to protect the bee population against infection, and to strengthen the comb when it is being built. Commercially, propolis can be collected from traps at the hive entrance, or by scraping.

CULINARY AND NUTRITIONAL VALUE

None.

CLAIMS AND FOLKLORE

Propolis was used as a medicine by the ancient Greeks, Romans, and Egyptians, and, in more modern times, in Europe, and during the Boer War in South Africa to treat fever and gangrene. Beekeepers often claim that the handling of propolis keeps the skin healthy and helps wounds heal quickly.

Extracts (e.g. ointments, creams) may be applied externally to treat small wounds, dermatitis, fungal infections, chilblains, and many other conditions. This would assume that propolis has antimicrobial and anti-inflammatory properties. Taken internally as tablets, capsules, lozenges, and sprays, propolis has been claimed to be effective against sore throats, colds, and chest (including tuberculosis), bladder, and kidney infections. Again, these actions may be associated with the antimicrobial and anti-inflammatory properties of propolis. Also, the suggestion has been made that propolis might stimulate the immune system of the body to protect against infection.

There are claims that propolis has no harmful side-effects (apart from relatively rare cases of allergy). It has also been claimed that bacteria, viruses, or fungi do not build up resistance to propolis. Apart from the antimicrobial actions of propolis, some studies have suggested that it may be able to scavenge free radicals, has antitumour properties, protects against gamma-irradiation, and regenerates bone, cartilage, and dental pulp.

EVIDENCE

A considerable number of scientific investigations have been carried out into the efficacy of propolis extracts – many in eastern Europe. These extracts have been shown to be effective against a number of Gram-positive bacteria (including the multidrug-resistant *Staphylococcus aureus*), rather than Gram-negative bacteria. Propolis was also shown to be active against *Mycobacterium tuberculosis*, the bacterium responsible for tuberculosis. There is also experimental evidence to support the action of propolis against fungi involved in skin infections and the types of viruses involved in colds and flu. Animal experiments have indicated the anti-inflammatory property of propolis. There is also support for the use of extracts as an antioxidant and local anaesthetic.

Propolis consists of resin (about 55%), wax (about 30%), essential oils (about 10%), pollen (about 5%), and other substances, but the composition depends on the source. The 'active' constituents are usually considered to be flavonoids and other phenolic compounds, known to have antibacterial and anti-inflammatory properties.

Without a doubt, studies so far do indicate possible therapeutic uses for propolis. However, more clinical studies are required to deal with standardization of constituents and dosage.

Bee products

Honey

ORIGIN

Honey is made from the nectar of flowers. The nectar is collected by the worker bee and stored in the crop or 'honey bag', where it is acted upon, during flight, by secretions from various glands. This leads to chemical changes in the nectar, which are continued in the hive. The resulting honey is deposited in the comb.

CULINARY AND NUTRITIONAL VALUE

It was used as a sweetening substance long before refined sugar – in bread, cakes, and sweetmeats – and, in some countries, is still used as such. Honey, or course, is consumed on its own, but also has many culinary uses, such as for curing ham and coating breakfast cereals. There are many different types of honey, depending on the flower source, and they vary in consistency and colour.

Fermented honey was used to make honey-wine (mead) in some ancient civilizations (e.g. Egypt, Greece, Rome, Scandinavia), and the beverage is still made today in various places.

Chemically, honey consists mainly of sugars: about 40% fructose, 35% glucose, and 4% other sugars, including sucrose (there is much more sucrose in the original nectar). The remainder of honey is about 18% water and numerous other substances, including a very small quantity of protein (< 0.26%) and minute amounts of minerals and vitamins (water soluble). Because minerals and vitamins are present in such small quantities, they can have very little nutritional significance. However, the presence of the easily absorbable glucose and fructose makes honey a rapid source of energy.

CLAIMS AND FOLKLORE

Many claims have been made for the medical use of honey. It is still used in cough mixtures. From early times it was applied as an antiseptic to skin sores and ulcers, and also applied to wounds by the ancient Egyptians, Assyrians, Romans, and Chinese; the Germans used it in the First World War. There have been many other applications, e.g. to induce sleep, and for diarrhoea, asthma, arthritis, and problems of the cardiovascular system.

EVIDENCE

Although it is difficult to find scientific evidence to support many of the claims made for honey, nevertheless, some of them have a reasonable basis. Its soothing (demulcent) property is useful in cough and cold mixtures. As applied to skin sores, wounds, and ulcers, the healing effect has been well recognized – a report in a fairly recent *British Journal of Surgery* confirms this. The effect is probably related to the antibacterial action of the high sugar concentration (a similar situation exists in jam).

A warning has been given about the possible presence of spores of *Clostridium botulinum* in honey. They germinate in older children and adults without giving problems, but may give rise in some infants to botulism. For this reason it has been recommended that honey should not be given to infants less than 1 year old.

Bee products

Pollen

ORIGIN

Pollen is produced in the stamens of the flower and consists of innumerable minute grains. It is the male element involved in the processes of pollination and fertilization. Pollen is collected by the worker bee from flowers, and carried as clumps, often multicoloured, on its hind legs. The clumps contain pollen from different flower species. For sale as a health food, it can be collected in traps at the entrance of the hive or as 'bee bread' within the hive.

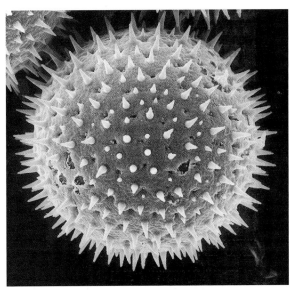

Mallow pollen grain, as seen with an electron microscope.

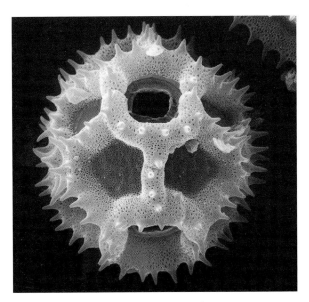

Dandelion pollen grain, as seen with an electron microscope.

CULINARY AND NUTRITIONAL VALUE

The chemical composition of pollen will depend on the flower species from which it is obtained but, in general terms, carbohydrates constitute up to 40%, protein 30%, and fatty substances 20%, and there are small quantities of substances such as vitamins (vitamin C may be present in quite a high amount), minerals, free amino acids, and flavonoids. Therefore, pollen is a balanced source of nutrients, but a large quantity would be required to play a significant part in the human diet, and this would be expensive.

CLAIMS AND FOLKLORE

A large number of claims have been made for the efficacy of pollen, including its value in dealing with anaemia, weight loss, enteritis, and colitis.

Pollen extracts are used to detect and provide immunity against certain human allergies. Consequently, consumers of pollen should be alert to allergic reactions.

EVIDENCE

There seems to be no real scientific support for the claims that have been made.

Bee products

Royal jelly

ORIGIN

Royal jelly is a salivary secretion of the worker bee. It is whitish in colour, has a doughy appearance, and possesses a slightly acidic flavour with a characteristic perfume. For the first 3 days all bee larvae are fed on royal jelly, but future queens continue to be nourished by it. They become much larger than workers, live longer, and are highly fertile. For these reasons it has been claimed that royal jelly could have a beneficial effect on human beings.

CULINARY AND NUTRITIONAL VALUE

The composition of royal jelly is 60–70% water, 10–15% carbohydrates, 4–8% fat, 11–18% protein, and a range of vitamins (pantothenic acid is present in relatively large amount) and minerals. Also present is hydroxydecenoic acid (2%). This acid has no nutritional value, but it has been claimed that it plays a part in other activities of royal jelly.

Therefore, royal jelly is well balanced as regards nutrients, but the intake often recommended by manufacturers is 150 mg per day (it may be raised to 300 mg). The nutrients thus supplied to an adult as part of the recommended daily intake are insignificant, e.g. 0.1–0.4% protein, 0.6% vitamin C, and 0.15–0.8% vitamin B_1. Royal jelly is a very expensive source of nutrients as far as the human is concerned.

CLAIMS AND FOLKLORE

Many claims have been made for the efficacy of royal jelly; e.g. treatment of hepatitis, eczema, and heart disease, prevention of colds, control of the ageing process, and removal of facial blemishes and wrinkles. It is said to have antibacterial qualities, possibly related to hydroxydecenoic acid.

EVIDENCE

Tests indicate that royal jelly has some slight antibacterial activity, but there is really no basis for the therapeutic claims.

Beverages *(see also guarana, p. 83)*

Coffee *Coffea arabica, C. canephora, C. liberica*

Family Rubiaceae

Coffee is made from the seeds (beans) of plants of the *Coffea* genus. There are a number of species of coffee plant that grow as shrubs or small trees. *C. arabica* provides about 90% of the world's coffee, with the remaining 10% coming mainly from *C. canephora* and *C. liberica*. The plants have small white flowers that give rise to crimson 'berries', each usually containing two 'beans'. After harvesting of the berries, the beans are extracted by one of two processes. In the wet process, the whole berry is first pulped and fermented in water; then the seeds are removed, the outer layer is stripped off mechanically, and the bean is dried. The dry process omits the soaking and fermentation, and the outer layers are removed mechanically after drying the berries. The wet process is considered to give the best coffee beans. Coffee beans are roasted before grinding, which brings out the aroma and flavour.

Coffee is drunk either as brewed coffee, with the ground beans being infused with water and the supernatant liquid drunk, or as instant coffee, where the infusion of coffee has been dried and can be reconstituted from the granules (freeze dried) or powder (spray dried) simply by adding water. Nutritionally both instant coffee and coffee made from the ground beans contain small amounts of protein and carbohydrate, such that a cup of either probably supplies 2–3 kcal if taken black. Coffee infusions and instant coffees both supply traces of B vitamins; nicotinic acid is present in appreciable amounts in both instant and brewed coffee, as it is released from the beans on roasting. Coffee also supplies potassium (between 60 and 100 mg per cup), with instant coffee tending to have higher levels than ground coffee due to the addition of anti-caking agents during manufacture.

The non-nutrient, biologically active compounds in coffee have been less extensively researched than those in tea (see below) but coffee contains a variety of polyphenolic compounds such as chlorogenic and caffeic acids that appear to have antioxidant properties. Roasting produces compounds called melanoidins, which also seem to act as free-radical scavengers (see p. xv).

Coffee contains the alkaloid caffeine (methylxanthine), which has stimulant and diuretic properties. A cup of ground coffee contains about 100–50 mg, instant coffee 60–70 mg, and decaffeinated coffee 1–5 mg.

Chicory *Cichorium intybus*

Family Compositae/Asteraceae

The ground root of the chicory plant has been used as a coffee substitute in times of shortage, either alone or added to coffee powder or essence. It has a bitter flavour and is caffeine free.

Dandelion *Taraxacum officinale*

Family Compositae/Asteraceae

The root of the dandelion plant has been used in a similar way to chicory, i.e. dried and ground to make a coffee substitute. The drink smells like coffee but has a bitter chicory flavour. Again it is caffeine free.

Beverages

Tea Camellia sinensis

Family Theaceae

All varieties of tea (except herbal teas) come from an evergreen plant, *Camellia sinensis*, which grows in tropical and subtropical climates. Tea has been used as a beverage in China for 2000–3000 years, and was introduced into Europe in the seventeenth century.

The majority of the tea harvest is made into black tea. This is produced by exposing the freshly picked leaves to air to promote a natural fermentation process, which results in a deep brown colour and the rich taste that is preferred in the USA, UK, Europe, and India. Green tea, popular in China and Japan, is the least fermented of teas – the leaves are steamed and retain their green colour. Oolong tea is a partially fermented tea. Tea may be blended with essential oils such bergamot or lemon, or mixed with other plant leaves to give different varieties, e.g. mint, chamomile, or jasmine, although sometimes these leaves may be used alone.

Nutritionally, true tea (*C. sinensis*), as drunk, is low in energy, and contains only traces of micronutrients. However, there are compounds in tea that are biologically active. Both black and green teas contain flavonoids that have antioxidant properties, i.e. help protect the body from the harmful effects of 'free radicals'. Many different types of flavonoids may be present in tea, but one group, the catechins, are particularly prevalent. In green tea the most prevalent catechin is epigallocatechin gallate, but the fermentation process in making black tea converts simple catechins into complex flavonoids called theaflavins and thearubigens (tannins) which, as well as having antioxidant functions, are responsible for the flavour and colour of the teas. In Oolong tea there is partial conversion of the flavonoids. Tea also contains caffeine. Levels of caffeine per cup of tea are less than instant coffee, and about half that of brewed coffee, and depend upon variables such as brewing time, water-to-leaf ratio, and water temperature. Moderate caffeine consumption is considered to be about 300 mg per day – equivalent to four to eight cups of brewed hot tea. Decaffeinated varieties of tea, containing about 5 mg of caffeine per cup, are available for people who are sensitive to the stimulant effects of caffeine.

Tea is the subject of a good deal of scientific interest at present. In test-tube studies bioflavonoids in tea appear to be more effective antioxidants than vitamin C, vitamin E, and beta-carotene, and there are suggestions that daily consumption of between two and five cups of tea may decrease the risk of chronic diseases such as heart disease, stroke, and cancer. Addition of milk does not seem to impair the absorption of the flavonoids. More work is necessary before these effects are confirmed.

The tannins in tea have been shown to reduce the amount of non-haem iron absorbed from foods that are eaten at the same meal. It has therefore been suggested that people with poor iron status should allow an hour between the end of a meal and drinking tea to minimize this effect.

Herbal teas

These are produced from a variety of plants, and may contain leaves, roots, flowers, and mixtures of spices and flavourings. They are generally lower in tannins than tea and taste less bitter. Some may be naturally rich in vitamin C, e.g. rose hip tea, while others may have the vitamin added. It is possible that some of these teas may contain other biologically active compounds with, for example, antioxidant properties, but there is no evidence of specific nutritional benefit from consumption.

Beverages

Maté *Ilex paraguariensis*

Family Aquifoliaceae

The green leaves of this plant (popular in South America) are prepared in a similar manner to tea and used to make a drink. The leaves contain about 2% caffeine, some of which is present in the infusion, and it has been suggested that it has both stimulant and diuretic effects. As pre-pared, the drink supplies about 13 kcal, a trace of protein and fat, and about 3 g of carbohydrate per 100 ml. It also supplies small amounts of calcium, iron, magnesium, and potassium, and tiny amounts of other minerals and trace elements.

Cola or kola nut *Cola acuminata or C. nitida*

Family Sterculiaceae

Cola nut is a native of tropical West Africa, but is also cultivated in that region, Brazil and Jamaica. In West Africa, particularly, it is a well known masticatory (chewing) stimulant, used to relieve fatigue and other conditions. It contains about 2% caffeine, which no doubt is responsible for its stimulant action. Products of cola may be found in health food stores.

Malted cereal drinks

These are drinks made from mixtures of cereals and other ingredients, such as milk and eggs, and are advocated as replacements for tea or coffee, or as bedtime drinks. Horlicks™ (TM = trade mark) and Ovaltine™ are advocated as nutritious drinks, and are fortified with calcium, iron, and a range of vitamins. The standard drinks require the addition of milk to make them, but instant varieties are now available that just require the addition of hot water. There are also flavoured varieties.

Some research has demonstrated that people, particularly the elderly, have a more 'restful' night after consuming these drinks, possibly due to the high carbohydrate content.

Table 10 Energy and nutrient content of two standard malted milk drinks (per 100 g of powder)

	Energy (kcal)	Protein (g)	Fat (g)	CHO[a] (g)	NSP (g)	Calcium (mg)	Iron (mg)	Vitamins					
								B_1 (mg)	B_2 (mg)	Folate (µg)	C (mg)	A (mg)	D (µg)
Horlicks	380	9.6	4.7	75.0	4.0	640	11.2	1.1	1.3	160	48	640	4
Ovaltine	360	7.3	1.9	78.3	N	800	28	1.4	1.6	N	120	625	5.0

[a]CHO, carbohydrates; NSP, non-starch polysaccharides; N, significant content but no information available.

Beverages

Barleycup™

This is an instant cereal drink that has no caffeine. It contains malted barley and rye with chicory and is caffeine free. It can be made with or without milk, and provides a range of nutrients as contained in the cereal (energy 244 kcal, protein 5.3 g, carbohydrate 55.6 g, and a trace of fat, per 100 g powder).

Mineral waters

Natural spring waters, especially those with strong flavours, have historically been ascribed health-giving properties. Spa towns where people went to 'take the waters' grew up around natural springs. Many of the original spring waters were rich in mineral salts and sulphur compounds, which may have had a diuretic or a purgative effect if drunk in reasonable quantity.

Today, vast quantities of bottled mineral or spring waters are sold. There are many named varieties, all of which make claims about taste and mineral content. They contain minerals such as sodium, potassium, and magnesium, and trace elements such as selenium, chromium, and others including, sometimes, small amounts of less desirable substances. Recently, calcium-fortified mineral water has come to the market in the UK. In the UK the composition and bacteriological safety of mineral waters is strictly controlled under The Natural Mineral Water, Spring Water and Bottled Drinking Water Regulations 1999.

Bottled waters have no special properties beyond supplying small amounts of minerals and trace elements in the diet, but because of the controls they are clean and low in contaminants such as nitrate and nitrite. Mineral waters should not be used to make up infant formulae as they contain too much sodium.

Bilberry, whortleberry, huckleberry, winberry
Vaccinium myrtillus

Family Ericaceae

ORIGIN AND CULTIVATION
Bilberry is found in Europe, Asia, and North America, growing on heaths, moors, and in acid, open woodlands. Because of its short stature, fruit collection is tedious and difficult, and therefore, it is not cultivated commercially but is often harvested locally. Its fruits, and to a lesser extent the leaves, are utilized.

PLANT DESCRIPTION
The plant is a low shrub, 20–60 cm (24 in) tall. It has green, angled twigs, bearing ovate and finely toothed leaves, 1–3 cm (1 in) long. The greenish pink flowers are solitary or in pairs. The fruits, about 6 mm in diameter, are pale red, ripening to blue–black in colour.

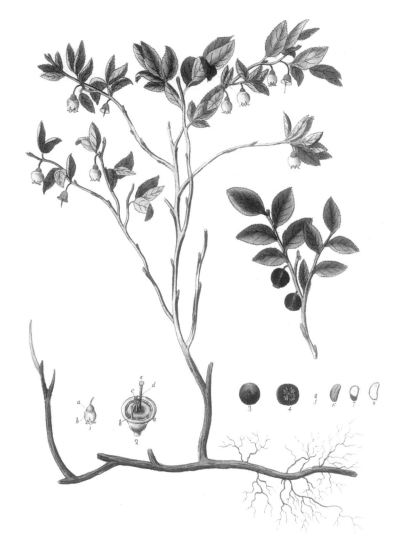

CULINARY AND NUTRITIONAL VALUE
The fruit is utilized in both fresh and dried conditions, and processed into jam, pastry products, juice, and wine. Its sugar content (7–14%) consists mainly of glucose and fructose. Vitamin C is present at 17 mg per 100 g.

CLAIMS AND FOLKLORE
Bilberry fruits and, to a lesser extent, leaves have played a part in traditional medicine. Fresh fruit is mildly laxative, but extracts of the dried fruit, because of their astringent and antiseptic activity, have been used for diarrhoea, dysentery, as a mouth wash, and as an antidiabetic agent.

EVIDENCE
Among other substances, the fruit contains anthocyanins (flavonoid-related), tannins, and flavonoids. There has been scientific investigation into the medical value and clinical use of bilberry products, for various microcirculation diseases (because of their possible blood capillary-strengthening activity) and for other vascular disorders. The fruit is approved in Germany but not the leaf.

Borage *Borago officinalis*

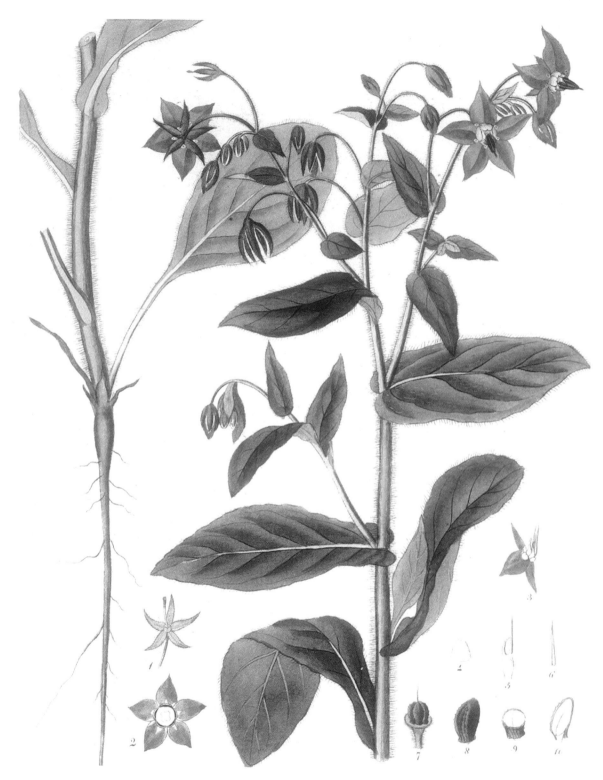

Borage

Family Boraginaceae

ORIGIN AND CULTIVATION

Borage is indigenous to dry, waste places of southern Europe, and naturalized in central, eastern, and western Europe. It has become established as a casual weed in eastern USA.

PLANT DESCRIPTION

The plant is an annual, 15–100 cm (40 in) in height, covered with coarse hairs and possessing wrinkled leaves. Its flowers are 1 cm ($\frac{1}{2}$ in) across, star-shaped, and bright blue. The tiny 'seeds' are brown to black in colour.

The parts used are the 'seeds' or nutlets (starflower oil), leaves, and flowers.

CULINARY AND NUTRITIONAL VALUE

The leaves, with a cucumber-like flavour, have been added to drinks, salads, soft cheese, and hors d'oeuvres. Alkaloids (of the pyrrolizidine type) are present, but in lower concentrations than in comfrey (*Symphytum*), for which human toxicity has been recorded. Nevertheless, ingestion should not be excessive.

The fresh flowers (said to be free of alkaloids) are included in salads or used as a garnish. They turn pink on contact with acids (lemon juice or vinegar). The flowers are also made into a syrup, or candied as cake decorations.

CLAIMS AND FOLKLORE

Borage has been part of European herbal medicine for centuries – the leaves and flowers steeped in wine were once said to dispel 'melancholy'. It has also been suggested that extracts: give relief to symptoms of rheumatism, colds, and bronchitis; can induce sweating and diuresis; increase breast milk production in women; act as a remedy in breast cancer and facial cancer; and improve dry skin conditions.

The seed oil (starflower oil) has come into prominence in recent years as a substitute for evening primrose oil (see p. 66). Starflower oil constitutes 28–38% of the seeds, and the oil contains 17–25% gamma-linolenic acid. The seed is therefore a richer source than that of evening primrose. As in the case of evening primrose, the oil serves as an important supplement of gamma-linolenic acid, a precursor of prostaglandins, which are necessary for the regulation of metabolic functions. The normal synthesis of gamma-linolenic acid from linoleic acid may be blocked or diminished in mammalian systems by various conditions, e.g. ageing and diabetes.

As in the case of evening primrose oil, starflower oil is said to be of value in treating atopic eczema, premenstrual syndrome, and as a preventative against heart disease and strokes.

EVIDENCE

There seems to be no scientific evidence to support the various suggested uses of borage, although the mucilage in the plant might act as an expectorant. Because of its alkaloids, the amount of borage ingested should be carefully controlled, particularly in pregnancy and lactation. Some countries regulate the use of borage.

The value of starflower oil is related to its gamma-linolenic acid content, although it has been stated that evening primrose oil is more biologically active. It is not approved in Germany.

Buchu *Barosma species*[1]

short buchu B. betulina; *long buchu* B. serratifolia; *ovate buchu* B. crenulata

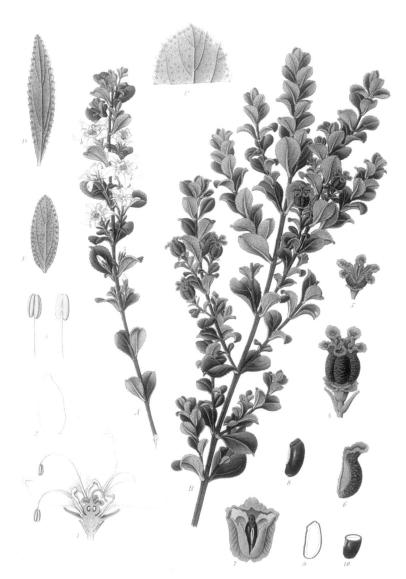

Family Rutaceae

ORIGIN AND CULTIVATION

Buchu is native to South Africa, where it grows wild but is also cultivated. Cultivation of the plant also takes place in other parts of the world. Of the three species, *Barosma betulina* is most commonly used in commerce. The English names applied to the different species refer to leaf features.

PLANT DESCRIPTION

The plant is a shrub growing to a height of 1–2.5 m (8 ft). Its leaves are studded with conspicuous oil glands and the flowers are white or pink. Buchu has a strong blackcurrant odour.

The leaves are the parts of the plant used in commerce.

[1] *Agathosma* has been used as a synonym for *Barosma.*

CULINARY AND NUTRITIONAL VALUE

Buchu essential oil is used as a component of artificial fruit flavours, particularly blackcurrant, and may be added to the alcoholic drink cassis.

CLAIMS AND FOLKLORE

The drug was originally used by the Hottentots of South Africa, and in the nineteenth century it appeared in the USA as a patent medicine. In modern herbal medicine it is usually prescribed as a diuretic and a urinary tract antiseptic.

EVIDENCE

A number of chemical constituents have been identified in buchu, but any therapeutic value is usually ascribed to its essential oil (1.0–3.5%) and, in particular, to a major component of the oil, namely diosphenol. There has been very little experimental work carried out on the therapeutic value of buchu, and any antiseptic action is probably very slight. There seems to be very little support for the drug in Germany. It is not recommended for use during pregnancy or lactation.

Burdock *Arctium lappa*

Family Compositae/Asteraceae

ORIGIN AND CULTIVATION

Burdock is a native of Europe and Asia. It is naturalized in the USA. The plant is cultivated in eastern Europe, Japan, China, and other countries in the East. *A. minus* is the chief American source of the root.

PLANT DESCRIPTION

It is a biennial or perennial that may grow to a height of 3 m (10 ft). The leaves are large, long-stalked, and ovate. Its flower head consists of a number of red–violet tubular florets, surrounded by many involucre bracts, terminating in stiff spiny hooks (a bur). The florets give rise to fawn 'seeds' (botanically speaking, these are fruits).

The taproot may attain 1.5 m (5 ft) in length, but for consumption a root of length 60–70 cm (28 in) and diameter 2.5–3 cm (1 in) is preferred.

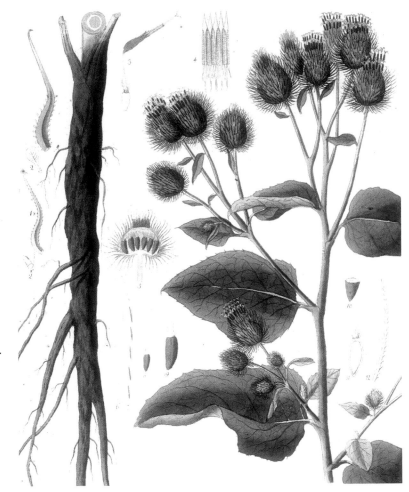

CULINARY AND NUTRITIONAL VALUE

The root (raw or cooked) is a common food in Asia, particularly Japan. It is generally considered to be safe, but could possibly cause a skin allergy. Sometimes the leaf stalks are scraped and cooked like celery.

CLAIMS AND FOLKLORE

Burdock has been used in herbal medicine in Europe since the Middle Ages; it has also played a part in Chinese medicine.

Decoctions or teas made from the seeds, roots, and leaves have been utilized to treat a wide range of ailments, including colds, catarrh, gout, and rheumatism, and also for the external treatment of various skin problems, such as acne and psoriasis.

Burdock has been included in cosmetic and toiletry preparations (e.g. hair tonics and anti-dandruff solutions) for its skin cleansing properties.

EVIDENCE

The root contains a wide range of compounds, with about 50% being composed of the polysaccharide inulin; the seed contains 15–30% oils and other compounds, and the leaf has a variety of substances. A number of animal experiments have indicated that burdock has mild antipyretic, antimicrobial (possibly due to the polyacetylenes present), diuretic, diaphoretic, laxative, and possibly antitumour properties. Seed extracts are said to show distinct hypoglycaemic activity in rats; fresh root juice seems to have antimutagenic properties. In spite of these experiments, the general feeling is that more investigations are required and that, at present, the scientific evidence does not support the herbal use of the plant; certainly this is the case in Germany.

Cases have been reported of adulteration of burdock with root of belladonna (*Atropa belladonna*). This has resulted in atropine poisoning.

Californian poppy *Eschscholzia californica*

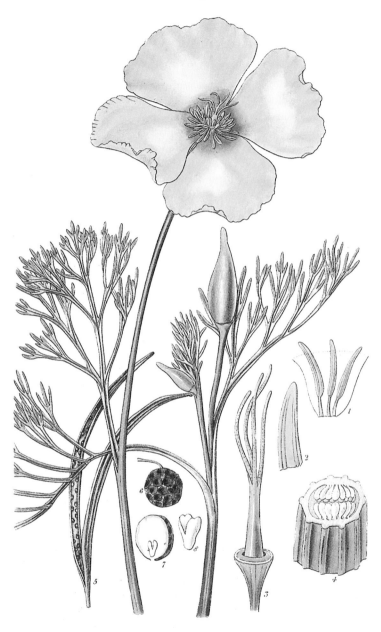

Family Papaveraceae

ORIGIN AND CULTIVATION

California poppy is native to western North America and grows wild in the coastal areas of south-west North America. It is frequently cultivated as a garden plant and is the state flower of California.

PLANT DESCRIPTION

The plant is an annual or short-lived perennial growing to a height of 20–60 cm (24 in), with finely divided blue–green leaves and orange, yellow, pink, or red flowers.

The aerial parts have been used in herbal medicine.

CULINARY OR NUTRITIONAL VALUE

None.

CLAIMS AND FOLKLORE

Californian poppy contains alkaloids and glycosides (flavone) and is mildly narcotic, but in no way like the highly narcotic opium poppy (*Papaver somniferum*). It was used by the native North Americans to treat toothache. Modern herbalists state that it is a diuretic, relieves pain, is antispasmodic, promotes perspiration, and is effective for nervous tension, insomnia, and incontinence (especially in children).

EVIDENCE

Some experimental work on Californian poppy has been carried out. There is no support for herbal use of the plant in Germany.

Carob, St John's bread, locust bean *Ceratonia siliqua*

Family Leguminosae/Fabaceae

ORIGIN AND CULTIVATION
Carob is native to southeastern Europe and western Asia, with a possible origin in Persia. It is cultivated in a number of Mediterranean countries (e.g. Greece, Spain, Italy, Cyprus, Israel), and trials of the plant have been carried out in California and Mexico. Selection of the crop has resulted in several superior cultivars (varieties).

PLANT DESCRIPTION
It is a dome-shaped evergreen tree growing to 15 m (50 ft) in height, with pinnate compound leaves consisting of 6–10 oval leaflets of leathery texture. The very small flowers are greenish or reddish and may be male, female, or have both types of sex organs. Its fruit is a fleshy, dark brown, oblong, flattened pod of up to 25 cm (10 in) long and 2.5 cm (1 in) wide, containing 10–12 black hard seeds within a soft, brownish pulp. The pod is the plant part of economic importance.

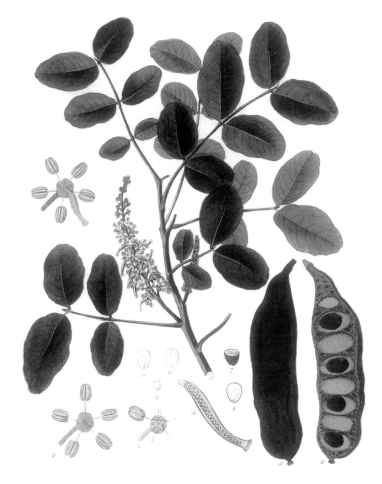

CULINARY AND NUTRITIONAL VALUE
Carob fruits were the 'locusts' eaten by John the Baptist. Because of their uniform size, the seeds were the original 'carat' weights used by jewellers.

The pod normally contains 40–50% sugars; sucrose and fructose are the major ones, but there are some other sugars present. In addition there is a wide range of chemical constituents, including proteins, amino acids, fats, and starch.

The seed contains protein, fats, tannins, a gum (galactomannan), and some other constituents.

Carob extract is obtained from the dried ripe pod (roasted or unroasted), and carob flour from the pulp or whole pod. The extract or flour are used, often as flavour constituents, in a very wide variety of foods, e.g. imitation chocolate, alcoholic and non-alcoholic beverages, meat products, biscuits, and confectionery. It is widely used in health food products. Carob is appreciated as a chocolate substitute by many who distrust true chocolate, presumably because of its fat and alkaloid contents.

The gum (galactomannan) extracted from the seed is used as a stabilizer for ice-cream, and as a thickener in many products, e.g. some foods, pharmaceuticals, detergents, and adhesives.

Crushed (kibbled) pods have often been included in animal feed, presumably because of their sweet flavour. For the same reason, there have been situations, at least in the past, when children bought these pods as confectionery.

CLAIMS AND FOLKLORE
In traditional medicine, the flour has been used to treat diarrhoea in babies, and catarrhal infections have been treated with decoctions of the pods.

EVIDENCE
No experimental evidence has been located.

Cat's claw *Uncaria tomentosa, U. guianensis*

Family Rubiaceae

ORIGIN AND CULTIVATION

The genus *Uncaria* contains about 35 species found throughout the tropics. Two species are presently of interest: *U. tomentosa* and *U. guianensis*. Both are found in South America.

PLANT DESCRIPTION

Both species are high-climbing, twining woody vines or lianas, with small curved spines on the stem.

The stem (and the root) bark is the source of herbal medicine.

CULINARY AND NUTRITIONAL VALUE

None.

CLAIMS AND FOLKLORE

Cat's claw has been used for a long time as a folk medicine in South America, where it is reputed to have value as a treatment for intestinal ailments (e.g. gastric ulcers, dysentery), gonorrhoea, and cancers (particularly of the urinary tract), and to be a wound healer and anti-inflammatory and antirheumatic agent.

The herb has begun to be utilized only relatively recently in Europe and the USA and, as in South America, is used, for treating various intestinal ailments, and as a possible AIDS treatment.

EVIDENCE

The chemistry of cat's claw has been well investigated, with emphasis on alkaloids and glycosides. A number of experiments have suggested that the herb might improve immunity in cancer patients, and may have antimutagenic properties, antihypertensive effects, a diuretic action, be a smooth muscle relaxant, and have local anaesthetic properties. However, there is a need for more controlled experiments. The material has a low toxicity.

Cat's claw is a good example of the necessity of standardizing preparations to the reputed active principles. Recent research has shown that *U. tomentosa* has two chemical types with respect to its alkaloids. One type, with predominantly pentacyclic alkaloids, reportedly has immunostimulant properties; the other, with predominantly tetracyclic alkaloids, can antagonize the therapeutic value of the first type. It is recommended that preparations of a mixture should contain less than 0.02% of the tetracyclic alkaloids.

Cayenne pepper *Capsicum frutescens, C. annuum*

Family Solanaceae

ORIGIN AND CULTIVATION
In pre-Columbian times, *Capsicum* was widely used in Central and South America, the Caribbean area, and Mexico. It is often stated that Columbus, on his return from the first voyage (1492), brought the plant back to Europe. From there it spread to Africa and Asia, very quickly becoming more important in those regions as a spice than 'black' or 'white' pepper (*Piper nigrum*).

PLANT DESCRIPTION
Because of its very long history of cultivation and human selection, many forms of *Capsicum* exist, and this makes classification difficult. Two species of *Capsicum* are usually recognized (*frutescens* and *annuum*).

Capsicum plants grow to a height of 0.5–1.5 m (5 ft), with ovate leaves and white to green flowers. The resulting fruits vary in size (being up to 30 cm (1 ft) in length), colour (yellow, red, brown), and pungency.

The dried fruit is the part used in herbal medicine.

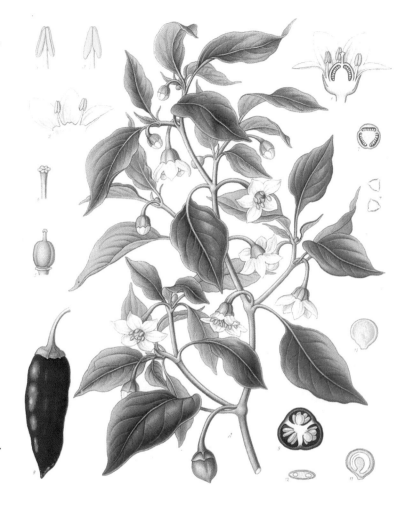

CULINARY AND NUTRITIONAL VALUE
Capsicum is of enormous importance as a vegetable and spice: sweet or bell peppers, paprika, chillies, tabasco, cayenne, and red pepper.

The fruit does not contain significant quantities of protein, fat, and sugars, but is a good source of carotenes (provitamin A) and vitamin C (up to 340 mg per 100 g of fresh material).

Extracts of the fruit are used to flavour and colour various foods and beverages, and also used in aerosols to deter 'muggers'.

CLAIMS AND FOLKLORE
Externally, *Capsicum* is applied to the skin, where it acts as an analgesic and rubefacient, producing a counter-irritant effect that deals with conditions such as rheumatism, arthritis, herpes, and some forms of neuralgia. Interestingly, *Capsicum* is included in mixtures placed in socks or stockings to keep the feet warm on cold days.

Internally, the drug has been employed as a stomachic, carminative, and gastrointestinal stimulant, also as a gargle for sore throats.

EVIDENCE
The pungent principles in *Capsicum* are capsaicin and related compounds (up to 1.5%), and these compounds are principally responsible for its drug action. There have been a number of human and animal investigations and some of its uses have been supported. The pungent principles can irritate delicate tissues and therefore can affect eyes. In certain individuals *Capsicum* may affect the lining of the gut; care should be taken with the drug during pregnancy and lactation. Both the external and internal uses of *Capsicum* are supported in Germany.

Celery seed *Apium graveolens*

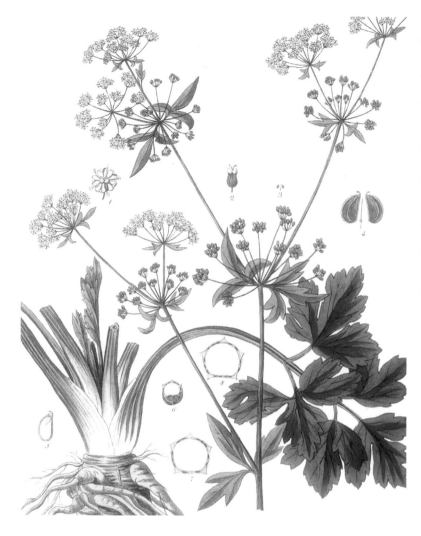

Family Umbelliferae/Apiaceae

ORIGIN AND CULTIVATION
Celery is a well known vegetable that has been cultivated for a long time, although wild forms are still found growing in moist places near the sea in Europe and Asia.

PLANT DESCRIPTION
The plant is a biennial, producing in its second year a tall flowering stem with terminal and axillary umbels of small, greenish white flowers, which develop into grey–brown-ridged 'seeds' (botanically speaking, the fruits), 1.5 mm in length.

Celery, both the whole plant and the seeds alone, have been used in herbal medicine. This entry concerns only the seed.

CULINARY AND NUTRITIONAL VALUE
The seeds may be used as a flavouring and in celery salt. Essential oil produced from the seed may be included as a flavouring in many food categories, including alcoholic and non-alcoholic beverages.

CLAIMS AND FOLKLORE
Late in the nineteenth century, various tonics were produced containing the juice of crushed celery seeds plus, very often, alcohol. Many claims have been made for the efficacy of celery seed as a diuretic (bladder and kidney complaints), sedative, carminative, and emmenagogue. It is also said to be useful in treating arthritis and rheumatism, and to have other uses, too.

EVIDENCE
Chemical analysis has revealed a considerable number of constituents in the seed. The essential oil contains limonene, selenine, phthalide compounds, and other substances. Although some animal experiments have been carried out, there is little evidence for its suggested therapeutic value.

The drug may cause dermatitis or allergies. It should be used with caution during pregnancy. The oil contains irritant substances, and, if used as a diuretic, might affect the urinogenital system. It is not supported in Germany.

Centaury *Centaurium erythraea syn. Erythraea centaurium*

Family Gentianaceae

ORIGIN AND CULTIVATION
Centaury grows in dry and sandy places in Europe, central Asia, and North Africa, and is naturalized in North America.

PLANT DESCRIPTION
The plant is a biennial, growing to a height of 15–24 cm (9 in), with a basal rosette of leaves. Its stems are branched, bearing clusters of pink or red flowers.

The whole plant is utilized in herbal medicine.

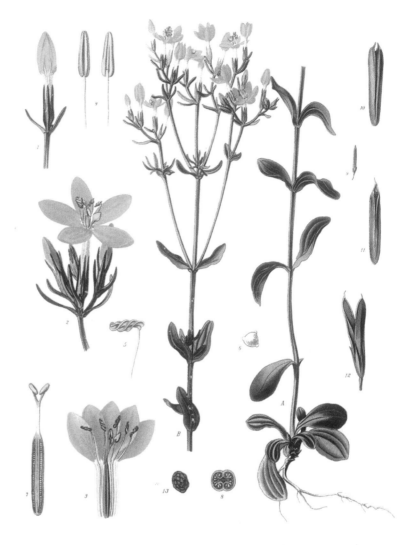

CULINARY AND NUTRITIONAL VALUE
Because it contains bitter substances, centaury is included in certain non-alcoholic and alcoholic (vermouth) beverages.

CLAIMS AND FOLKLORE
Centaury is reported to have had a number of herbal uses. It has been given as a bitter tonic to increase gastric secretions, it has been used for the relief of dyspeptic discomfort and loss of appetite, and it has been included in cosmetic and toilet preparations for alleged soothing and astringent properties. There have also been claims that the herb has sedative, antipyretic, and other actions.

EVIDENCE
Centaury contains bitter glycosides, alkaloids, phenolic acids, and other substances. There is very little experimental work concerning the efficacy of this herb, although its bitter constituents support its use as an appetite stimulant.

Because there is a lack of knowledge about its effects, it is not recommended for use during pregnancy and lactation.

Cereals

Overview

Cereal grains are important staple foods providing substantial amounts of energy, protein, and micronutrients for much of the world's population. The main cereals consumed are wheat, rice, oats, maize (corn), wild rice (*Zizania aquatica*), rye, barley, sorghum, and millets, and these are all part of the grass family of plants (Gramineae/Poaceae). Triticale (× *Triticosecale*) is a wheat–rye hybrid. Buckwheat (*Fagopyrum esculentum*), quinoa (*Chenopodium quinoa*), and amaranth (*Amaranthus* species), while not true cereals, are seeds of plants that have become increasingly available in recent years and are known as pseudo-cereals.

The cereal 'grain' is the fruit of the plant, which is harvested, separated from the chaff and straw, and processed to a greater or lesser extent to produce acceptable staple foods. Cereal grains supply a range of nutrients in the diet, including starch, protein, fat, dietary fibre (insoluble and soluble non-starch polysaccharides), and some vitamins (B vitamins and E) and minerals.

The nutrients in cereals are distributed unevenly throughout the grain. The grain is usually described in terms of the outer bran layer (pericarp, testa, and aleurone layer), the flour or endosperm, and germ (scutellum and embryo).

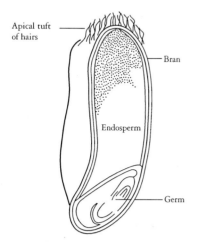

A vertical section of a wheat grain.

The bran is rich in dietary fibre, B vitamins, and minerals; the endosperm is rich in starch and protein; and the germ is rich in unsaturated fat, vitamins B and E, and minerals.

In all cereals starch is the main carbohydrate, making up a large amount of the endosperm and providing, on average, 75% of the weight of the grain. The protein content of cereal grains varies from 3.4 to 15%, with whole-wheat and oats at the top of the range and rice at the lower end. Protein quality also varies, as cereals tend to have low amounts of certain essential amino acids, typically lysine. This is generally corrected for in most diets by eating complementary foods with the cereals that supply the missing lysine, e.g. bread and cheese, breakfast cereal and milk, rice and peas or beans. The proteins in the pseudo-cereals (buckwheat, quinoa, and amaranth) have a higher lysine content than the major cereals, and some other cereal cultivars (e.g. maize varieties) have also now been bred to provide a higher lysine content.

The fat content of most cereals is low, about 2–4%, with the exception of some types of oats and maize for which the level may be as high as 10%. Cereal fat is liquid at room temperature and therefore better described as oil. The major fatty acids in cereals are oleic (monounsaturated), linoleic (polyunsaturated), and palmitic (saturated), with the unsaturated acids usually making up at least 75% of the total fat. The fat may be distributed throughout the endosperm, as in oats, or concentrated in the germ of the seed. Maize germ is particularly high in fat, and this cereal is an important source of cooking oil production.

The vitamin and mineral content of cereal products varies with the degree of processing of the grain. As the vitamins are found largely in the germ and outer layers of cereals, removal of these on milling will reduce the amounts left in the food as eaten. This is also the case for the minerals and trace elements present, e.g. potassium, calcium, iron, zinc, copper, magnesium, and manganese. However, these minerals may not be readily available to the body anyway, as they are bound to the phytates in the grain. Some processes, such as fermentation and leavening in bread-making, and malting of barley, improve the availability of the minerals.

Cereals may be processed to varying extents; e.g. wheat flour may be made from the whole grain, or increasing amounts of the bran and germ may be removed to supply brown or white flour. White flour typically contains only 20–50% of the dietary fibre, vitamins, and minerals of whole-grain bread, and in some countries fortification of white flour is mandatory, in an attempt to replace the lost nutrients.

Many claims have been made for the health benefits of eating cereal foods, and the current guidelines for a healthy diet in most countries recommend that starchy foods such as cereal provide a high proportion of the energy in the diet. In the USA, the Food and Drug

Cereals

Administration allows claims to be made for the health benefits of consuming wholegrains in relation to both cancer prevention and heart disease. For example:

- Low-fat diets rich in fiber-containing grain products, fruits, and vegetables may reduce the risk of some types of cancer, a disease associated with many factors.

- Diets low in saturated fat and cholesterol and rich in fruits, vegetables, and grain products that contain some types of dietary fiber, particularly soluble fiber, may reduce the risk of heart disease, a disease associated with many factors.

In the UK the Joint Health Claims Initiative (JHCI) has also sanctioned a generic claim – 'People with a healthy heart tend to eat more wholegrain foods as part of a healthy lifestyle'.

There are also specific health benefits claimed for certain cereals such as oats, rye, and barley, which will be considered below.

Certain cereals may cause adverse reactions in some people because of their sensitivity to proteins in the grain. The most important of these is gluten-sensitive enteropathy, or coeliac disease. Gluten is the main protein complex in wheat bread, and gliadins, (components of this protein), together with similar protein fractions in rye and barley (and possibly oats), cause reactions in the lining of the small intestine which destroy the absorptive surface of the gut. In young children or severe cases, vomiting, diarrhoea, and malabsorption will result, although in older children and adults the gastrointestinal symptoms are often slight or absent. The person may simply complain of excess flatulence or intermittent abdominal pain, and constipation is not uncommon. However, damage is still being done to the small intestine, and there may be hidden malabsorption of certain vitamins and minerals which can result in anaemia or bone disease in the long term. There is an associated skin disease, dermatitis herpetiformis, which also results in changes in the gastric mucosa. The treatment for both of these conditions is a gluten-free diet. This requires complete avoidance of the cereals containing gluten and gliadin-like protein fractions, i.e. wheat, barley, triticale, and rye. There is some controversy over the need to eliminate oats from the diet, as some people appear to be intolerant to this while others are not. Buckwheat, despite the name, is not a true cereal and does not contain gluten. Gluten-free foods are discussed in the next section.

There are people without coeliac disease or dermatitis herpetiformis who appear not to tolerate wheat or some other cereals, and find that either adverse gastrointestinal symptoms such as irritable bowel syndrome or other signs of food intolerance such as asthma, eczema, or migraine are alleviated by removing these from the diet.

Gluten-free foods

These foods do not contain wheat, rye, triticale, or barley flours. The main protein complex in wheat is gluten and small fractions of this complex – gliadins – cause an adverse reaction in sensitive people. Rye also contains some gluten, and there are similar protein fractions in barley (hordein) and oats (avenin).

Some cereals – rice, maize, sorghum, and millets – are naturally free of the harmful proteins, since neither they nor the pseudo-cereals – buckwheat, quinoa, and amaranth – contain any gluten. Mixtures of these grains, sometimes with other ingredients such as potato flour, are used to produce gluten-free flours that can then be made into breads, cakes, and biscuits. Ready-made bread, cakes, and biscuits are also available, as are bread mixes. Bread made from gluten-free flours is not the same as ordinary bread, because the fermentation of gluten is responsible for the elasticity of the dough and hence the structure of the loaf. Most gluten-free bread is made from wheat starch, which is flour from which the gluten has been removed plus additives to enable the bread to rise. Milk or other proteins may be added to the flours to improve the texture and colour of the baked products, and these foods should therefore not be regarded as low-protein products.

Traces of gluten may remain in wheat starch, and some people are intolerant to even small amounts. (The World Health Organization's *Codex Alimentarus* defines a product as being gluten free if the nitrogen content does not exceed 0.05 g per 100 g flour.)

Cereals

Wheat and wheat products

Family Gramineae/Poaceae

Wheat types are characterized as hard or soft depending on the milling characteristics of the grain. Hard wheats yield coarse gritty flour which is easily sifted, while soft wheats give very fine flour, which is difficult to sieve as the particles stick to each other and clog the sieve. Flours are also characterized as strong or weak according to the amount and properties of the gluten-forming proteins. Strong flours contain more gluten-forming proteins and are used mainly for bread-making. Hard wheat usually makes strong flour – but not always. Weak flours have less protein and are used to make cakes and biscuits.

For example, the hard wheat *Triticum aestivum* is used to make strong bread flour that forms elastic gluten when water is added and the dough kneaded. During the bread-making process this holds the carbon dioxide produced by fermentation of the added yeast, to give a leavened loaf. Much of the hard wheat suitable for bread-making is produced in the USA and Canada, while wheats grown in the UK tend to produce flour more suitable for cakes and pastries. The Chorleywood bread process, developed in the 1960s, enabled more UK-grown wheat to be incorporated into bread. One effect of this has been to reduce the amount of selenium (see p. xx) in the UK diet. Selenium is incorporated into foods from the soil on which the crop is grown, and soils in the UK are lower in selenium than those in Canada and the USA. The low selenium content of UK wheat is likely to affect people eating a vegan diet most, as lacto-ovo vegetarians and omnivores can obtain the mineral from animal sources.

Durum wheat (*Triticum durum*) is another hard wheat that has even more protein than bread wheat, but because the structure of the protein is different it does not make such good bread. When milled it breaks into semolina, a coarse flour which is used to make pasta, couscous, and bulgar.

Wholewheat products supply significant amounts of dietary fibre, mainly of the insoluble form, which helps prevent constipation. As progressively more of the outer layers and the germ of the wheat are removed on milling to flour, so the content of dietary fibre and the mineral and vitamin content of the flour is reduced. White bread in the UK is normally fortified to replace the nutrients lost on milling – calcium, iron, vitamin B_1, and niacin are added. Table 11 demonstrates that wheat bran is a good source of other nutrients as well as dietary fibre (non-starch polysaccharides).

Flours may be milled in different ways. Stoneground flours are produced by grinding the grain between two stones, one stationary and the other moving. The texture of the flour is controlled by the distance between the stones and by the sieving of the flour produced. Most flour is now produced by roller-milling.

Wholemeal flours are made from the whole grain, including the bran and germ, and therefore retain all the nutrients from the grain. In the USA the preferred term is wholewheat or Graham flour, and in India a product that is almost wholegrain, called *atta*, is produced for making chapattis. The proportion of the whole grain that remains after milling is known as the extraction rate. Wholegrain flours have an extraction rate of 100%, brown flours between 85 and 98%, and white flours from 70 to 85%. Granary flour contains whole or cracked grains.

White flour may have chemical agents added to bleach the natural pigment in the endosperm, and other materials may be added to facilitate the bread-making process. Unbleached flours do not contain these additives.

Flours may be 'plain', or have raising agents such as baking powder (sodium bicarbonate and sodium bitartrate) added to lighten the products made with them. Such 'self-raising' flours therefore contain more sodium.

Table 11 Changes in energy and nutrient intake with milling (per 100g of product)

	Energy (kcal)	Protein (g)	Fat (g)	CHO[a] (g)	NSP (g)	Calcium (mg)	Iron (mg)	Vitamin B_1 (mg)	Vitamin B_2 (mg)	Folate (µg)
Wheat grain	339	13.7	2.5	71.1	N	34	3.5	0.42	0.12	N
Wholemeal flour	310	12.7	2.2	63.9	9	38	3.9	0.47	0.09	60
White flour	341	11.5	1.4	75.3	3.1	15[b]	1.5[b]	0.10[b]	0.15	22
Bran	206	14.1	5.5	26.8	36.4	110	12.9	0.90	1.38	260

[a] CHO, carbohydrates; NSP, non-starch polysaccharides; N, no value available but likely to have a significant amount.
[b] Unfortified. Fortified flour contains about 140 mg calcium, 2.0 mg iron, and 0.32 mg vitamin B_1.

Cereals

Semolina is the coarsely ground endosperm of durum wheats, and is used to make pasta and couscous. Pasta was traditionally made by mixing the semolina with water and kneading it to a dough, which could be extruded in a press to form thin sheets that were cut into strips and allowed to dry. It is now more than 50 years since machines with specially shaped dies were invented that allow different shapes such as spirals and bows to be extruded. The processes by which pasta is produced modifies the starch contained in the wheat in such a way that it is digested slowly and results in a slow rise in blood sugar levels after a meal; i.e. it is said to be a food with a 'low glycaemic index' (see p. xv).

Couscous is produced by making a paste with the semolina and water, and drying and grinding it to a similar consistency to very coarse semolina, in which form it has excellent keeping properties.

Bulgar consists of parboiled whole, or crushed, partially de-branned wheat grains, which are used as a substitute for rice. In the Old Testament this was referred to as *arisah* and prepared by boiling wheat grains until tender, then spreading them out in the sun to dry. The outer bran layers were removed by sprinkling with water and rubbing by hand, and the grains were then cracked using stones or a crude mill. It is now prepared commercially by rather more sophisticated methods. It has been suggested that the parboiling process retains the B vitamins (especially thiamin, niacin, and riboflavin) in the cereal, as these are distributed throughout the grain before the outer layers are removed.

WHEATBRAN

This is the outer layer of the wheat grain, and contains some starch and protein as well as about 40% by weight dietary fibre (slightly less if expressed as non-starch polysaccharides). Coarse bran in particular has been shown to hold water in the intestines and prevent constipation. If the bran is ground to a finer powder this effect is less marked. Addition of raw bran to an otherwise low-fibre diet is not the best way to increase dietary fibre intake, as the bran also contains significant amounts of phytate, a phosphorus-containing compound that binds minerals such as iron, zinc, and calcium. In bread the actions of the yeast and the cooking process release the minerals, but if raw bran is added to the diet these nutrients may not be absorbed.

WHEATGERM

When wheat is milled, various fractions are milled off. Wheatgerm is the fraction that contains most of the embryo (the part of the grain that would develop into a new plant if it were allowed to grow) and the layer separating this from the starchy endosperm. Wheatgerm is rich in protein, contains most of the (polyunsaturated) fat of the grain, and contains useful amounts of thiamin, folate, vitamin E, magnesium, iron, and zinc per 100 g of food. However, most people only consume a small amount of it.

SPELT WHEAT *Triticum spelta*

Spelt wheat grain and flour made from it are sold in health food outlets and some supermarkets. It is cultivated in Italy, France, Spain, USA, and Germany. Spelt wheat is a 'hulled' wheat; when threshed, the grain is still enclosed within hulls (part of the chaff) and these are removed during milling (similar to barley, oats, rice) to give the groat. The 'hulled' character, as far as modern wheats are concerned, may be regarded as primitive.

Views are mixed concerning the origin of the wheat. It is often said to have originated in the Near East (possibly Iran), but another view is that Europe is the centre of origin. Its arrival could have been in the Bronze Age.

From a nutritional point of view it is similar to bread wheat, although it is said to be easier to digest and to have a better taste. There are also claims that individuals with certain allergies to bread wheat can consume spelt wheat. Nevertheless, it should not be assumed that spelt wheat can be eaten by people with coeliac disease.

Cereals

KAMUT

Kamut is a brand of durum wheat (*Triticum durum*) with an apparently interesting history. Seeds were introduced into the USA from Egypt in recent times and used to develop the kamut crop. Grain, flour, and other products of this wheat are available in health food outlets.

The grain seems to be somewhat nutritionally superior to other wheats, particularly in relation to its protein content. It is said that the food products of the wheat have a mild nutty flavour, and it is also claimed that they do not cause as many allergic reactions as ordinary wheat. Kamut wheat should not be eaten by people with coeliac disease.

Oats Avena sativa

Family Gramineae/Poaceae

Oats are a cool-season crop growing mainly in northern Europe (Russia is the main producer), probably since 1000 BC. Grown mainly as an animal feed, the grain has seen an upsurge in use as a human foodstuff as various beneficial properties have been ascribed to it. After threshing the hulls are removed by milling, leaving the whole of the groat, which is usually used in human foodstuffs. Oatmeal, or 'pinhead oats', is produced by cutting the groat into sections, and may be used for making porridge and in cakes, biscuits, etc. Flaked or rolled oats are the most familiar form, and are produced by passing steam-cooked groats or pieces of groat between heavy flaking rollers. The steam process completes the inactivation of enzymes in the oats that can cause rancid flavours due to breakdown of fat, and also helps gelatinize the starch so that less cooking is needed at home. Thin, fine flakes made from pinhead require less cooking than the large, thick jumbo oat which result from large whole groats. Oat bran is produced by removing most of the endosperm, leaving the pericarp, which contains a high proportion of non-starch polysaccharides (dietary fibre). Oat flours resulting from this process are used to make extruded breakfast cereals. Rolled oats (or whole groats) may be used in muesli-type cereals and cooked to make porridge.

Of the cereals, oats have the highest level of both protein (up to 20%, according to cultivar) and fat (5–9%). The fat in oats is also mainly unsaturated and the cereal supplies a range of B vitamins. Over recent years it has been demonstrated that consumption of rolled oats (in amounts of about 125–150 g per day), or oat bran in smaller amounts, will lower blood cholesterol levels, especially in people who have high initial levels. It is thought that the beta-glucan part of the non-starch polysaccharides in oats is largely responsible for this effect. In the USA the Food and Drug Administration have allowed a health claim to this effect; a sample claim would be:

> Diets low in saturated fat and cholesterol that include 3 g of soluble fiber from whole oats per day may reduce the risk of heart disease. One serving of this whole-oats product provides x g of this soluble fiber.

In 2004 the JHCI in the UK allowed a similar claim:

> The inclusion of oats as part of a diet low in saturated fat and a healthy lifestyle can help reduce blood cholesterol.

Table 12 Energy and nutrient content of oatmeal (per 100g)

	Energy (kcal)	Protein (g)	Fat (g)	CHO[a] (g)	NSP (g)	Calcium (mg)	Iron (mg)	Vitamin B_1 (mg)	Vitamin B_2 (mg)	Folate (µg)
Oatmeal	401	12.4	8.7	72.8	6.8	44	4.1	0.50	0.10	60[b]

[a] CHO, carbohydrates; NSP, non-starch polysaccharides.
[b] An estimate.

Cereals

Oats do not contain gluten per se, but they do have protein fractions similar to those that cause problems in patients with coeliac disease. This remains controversial, but recent opinion suggests that oats can be included in the diets of most people with this disorder.

Barley *Hordeum vulgare*

Family Gramineae/Poaceae

Barley is a cereal crop that is cultivated widely. It tolerates most conditions, including cold, salt, and, if the humidity is low, high temperatures. Grown in most of Europe, Canada, the USA, Asia, China, the Near East, and India, as well as on the Mediterranean fringe of North Africa and Ethiopia, its main use is for animal food. It is also used to make malt and used as human food – mainly as 'pearl' or 'pot' barley. Barley flour is produced by grinding the milled barley and was commonly used to make bread in Roman times. However, this bread is usually flat and heavy as barley does not contain gluten-producing proteins. Although barley does not form gluten per se it does contain gliadin-like proteins, which mean that it is not suitable for people who need a gluten-free diet.

Pearl and pot barley consist of the inner layers of the grain only, as the outer layers are removed on milling. This means that only traces of the vitamins, minerals, and non-starch polysaccharides in the whole grain remain in the finished product, but it is a useful starchy addition to soups and stews. Beta-glucans in the endosperm of barley may have similar effects to those in oats – but so little barley is usually eaten that the effects are insignificant.

It is claimed that several beverages made from barley have beneficial effects. Barley water is made by soaking and boiling pot or pearl barley and straining off the liquid, which may then be flavoured with orange or lemon before drinking. The beneficial effect is possibly that it provides an easily absorbed source of carbohydrate when people are unable to eat food. A coffee substitute, Barleycup (see p. 19), is made from freeze-dried extracts of roasted barley, mixed with rye and chicory. This supplies more energy, carbohydrate (including some soluble non-starch polysaccharides), and sodium than instant coffee, but is caffeine-free and contains less potassium

Malt extract is a by-product of the brewing industry. Barley grains are germinated to produce enzymes, dried, lightly cooked, and the culms (sprouts) removed. Water is added to the crushed malt, and the enzymes ferment the starch in the grain to sugars. In brewing the sugars will then be fermented to alcohol by the addition of yeast.

Malt extracts are made from the residue of the sprouted grains by concentrating and standardizing the water content. The extracts contain the partially digested starch, resulting in a high maltose (39–42% of the product) and maltotriose (about 10–15%) content. The remaining carbohydrate consists of small amounts of glucose and some complex polysaccharides. As well as being used to flavour breads, and other baked goods such as bagels, malt extract is sometimes used as a 'tonic' – it contains a range of B vitamins and a small amount of vitamin C (about 10 mg per 100 g). Some malt extracts are supplemented with cod-liver oil, which supplies omega-3 fatty acids and vitamins A and D. Typical fat-soluble vitamin contents per 100 g of malt extract with cod-liver oil might be 2245 µg of vitamin A, 30 µg of vitamin D, and 300 µg of vitamin E.

Table 13 Energy and nutrient content of barley (per 100 g)

	Energy (kcal)	Protein (g)	Fat (g)	CHO[a] (g)	NSP (g)	Calcium (mg)	Iron (mg)	Vitamin B_1 (mg)	Vitamin B_2 (mg)	Folate (µg)
Barley										
wholegrain	301	10.6	2.1	64.0	14.8	50	6.0	0.31	0.10	50
pearl	360	7.9	1.7	83.6	N	20	3.0	0.12	0.05	20

[a] CHO, carbohydrates; NSP, non-starch polysaccharides; N, present in significant amount but no data available.

Cereals

Table 14 Energy and nutrient content of malt extract (per 100 g)

	Energy (kcal)	Protein (g)	Fat (g)	CHO[a] (g)	NSP (g)	Calcium (mg)	Iron (mg)	Vitamin B_1 (mg)	Vitamin B_2 (mg)	Folate (µg)
Malt extract	325	4.4	Tr	74.3	–	14	0.26	0.26	0.77	–

[a] CHO, carbohydrates; NSP, non-starch polysaccharides; Tr, trace; –, no value available.

Rye Secale cereale

Family Gramineae/Poaceae

Rye is a cereal grown in colder parts of northern and central Europe and Russia. It is mainly used for animal feed, but is also used to make breads and crispbreads. Rye contains gluten-forming proteins and is therefore not suitable for gluten-free diets.

The dough produced by rye flour is less elastic than wheat dough, and the breads therefore tend to be heavy and flat unless the rye flour is mixed with wheat to aid leavening and lighten the colour. Rye bread may be made by standard bread-making methods, or by sourdough processes whereby starter doughs containing lactic acid are added to the flours. These give a distinctive flavour to the dough. Pumpernickel is a dark rye bread made from coarse grain by a sourdough process, with a long baking time that ensures that it keeps for a long time.

Rye crispbreads are made from wholemeal or flaked rye, mixed with water or milk. The dough may be fermented with yeast to make brown crispbread, or unfermented (white crispbread), The nutrient value of crispbreads depends on the ingredients, but will be similar to the whole grain if this was used. They are commonly regarded as low energy foods – partly because they are light. However, weight for weight, crispbreads are more energy and nutrient dense than bread because of their low water content.

Table 15 Energy and nutrient content of rye and rye products (per 100 g)

	Energy (kcal)	Protein (g)	Fat (g)	CHO[a] (g)	NSP (g)	Calcium (mg)	Iron (mg)	Vitamin B_1 (mg)	Vitamin B_2 (mg)	Folate (µg)
Rye	335	14.8	2.5	69.8	–	33	2.7	–	–	–
Rye bread	219	8.3	1.7	45.8	4.4	80	2.5	0.29	0.05	24
Rye crispbread	321	9.4	2.1	70.6	11.7	45	3.5	0.28	0.14	35

[a] CHO, carbohydrates; NSP, non-starch polysaccharides; –, no value available.

Rice Oryza sativa

Family Gramineae/Poaceae

Rice is a cereal that needs to be grown in water to give the best yields. It is the second most important staple crop in the world; most of the yield (about 96%) is used as the main food in the country of growth and never enters the world markets. When harvested, rice grains are enclosed in a hull, which is removed in the first stage of milling to produce brown or wholegrain rice. Brown rice contains all the minerals and vitamins of the grain as well as some dietary fibre and it is therefore a useful food, despite needing longer cooking times than the more highly milled white rice which has the germ and bran removed. White rice is still a useful source of carbohy-

Cereals

drate and energy; protein content is not high but it has a good pattern of amino acids. White rice is low in thiamin and other B vitamins, and in countries where white rice is the staple, supplemented by few other foods, has led to the development of the thiamin deficiency disease, beriberi. This was commonly seen in Japanese prisoners of war during the Second World War. Parboiling of rice prior to milling it to white rice distributes the vitamins and minerals through the grain, and has been used as a preventative measure.

Rice is often classified by grain length, and described as long, medium, or short grain. The different types have different culinary uses; long grain rice is usually boiled in water and eaten with savoury dishes; short grain rice is used for milk puddings. In Mediterranean cooking rice with round short grains is used for making 'risotto'.

Rice bran is commonly used as animal feed, but some is now also sold as a source of dietary fibre for those who cannot tolerate wheat.

Wild rice (*Zizania aquatica*) is not strictly rice, but rather the seed of an aquatic grass that grew wild in lakes in the north of the USA and south of Canada. The grain is now grown for the world market, and provides elongated shiny black–brown grains that have a nutty flavour and chewy texture when cooked. The grain is nutritious, having a higher protein and B vitamin content than cereals generally, but it is usually eaten in smaller quantities.

Rice and wild rice are both gluten free.

Table 16 Energy and some nutrients (per 100 g of uncooked rice)

	Energy (kcal)	Protein (g)	Fat (g)	CHO[a] (g)	NSP (g)	Calcium (mg)	Iron (mg)	Vitamin B$_1$ (mg)	Vitamin B$_2$ (mg)	Folate (µg)
Rice										
brown	357	6.7	2.8	81.3	1.9	10	1.4	0.59	0.07	49
white	361	6.5	1	86.8	0.5	4	0.5	0.08[b]	0.02	20[b]
wild	357	14.7	1.1	74.9	N	21	2.0	0.12	0.26	95
Rice cakes	387	8.2	2.8	81.5	N	11.6	1.49	0.06	0.17	21

[a] CHO, carbohydrates; NSP, non-starch polysaccharides; N, no value available but likely to have significant amount.
[b] An estimate.

Maize Zea mays

Family Gramineae/Poaceae

The oldest remains of maize (corn) have been found in Mexico, dating back to about 5500 BC. It has proved a very adaptable crop and is now cultivated in every type of region, from tropical to temperate areas and in almost every continent.

Although most of the grain produced is used as animal feed, nevertheless, it is important in the human diet (e.g. popcorn, sweetcorn, porridges, hominy, Italian 'polenta', tortillas). Sweetcorn is the 'wet' form, and may be eaten boiled or baked on the cob or as fresh or frozen kernels. The dried cereal is often consumed as 'popcorn', a snack that in its pure form is relatively filling and low in energy. However, butter and sugar added to it increase the energy and it is also often salted, thus increasing sodium intake. Milling of the dried kernels removes bran and germ, and grinding will reduce the endosperm to cornflower, which is used as a thickening agent and in baking.

Generally speaking, the distribution of nutrients in the grain follows the pattern described for cereals previously. However, some special points can be made. The germ contains a large amount (25–50%) of a highly polyunsaturated oil (60% linoleic acid) – important as a cooking oil. Tortillas are a well known food item in Mexico and Central America, and elsewhere. In maize, the vitamin niacin is in a bound form. Deficiency of niacin, coupled with a low-protein diet, leads to the disease pellagra. To release niacin for human absorption the maize is treated with lime.

Yellow corn contains pigments, one of which is beta-carotene, a precursor of vitamin A in the human body.

Maize and its products are all suitable for gluten-free diets.

Cereals

Table 17 Energy and nutrient content of maize and its products (per 100 g)

	Energy (kcal)	Protein (g)	Fat (g)	CHO^a (g)	NSP (g)	Calcium (mg)	Iron (mg)	Vitamin B$_1$ (mg)	Vitamin B$_2$ (mg)	Folate (µg)
Sweetcorn kernels (fresh)	93	3.4	1.8	16.6	1.5	3	–	0.16	0.05	41
Maize grits	362	8.7	0.8	77.7	N	4	–	0.13	0.04	–
Cornflour	354	0.6	0.7	92	0.1	15	1.4	Tr	Tr	Tr

^{a} CHO, carbohydrates; NSP, non-starch polysaccharides; –, no value available; N, no value available but likely to have significant amount; Tr, trace.

Millet *Eleusine coracana, Pennisetum typhoideum, Panicum miliaceum*

Family Gramineae/Poaceae

There are a number of millet species, e.g. finger millet (*Eleusine coracana*), pearl millet (*Pennisetum typhoideum*), common millet (*Panicum miliaceum*), and other species. They are small seeded cereals (sorghum (*Sorghum bicolor*) has larger seeds). Generally speaking, the millets can be cultivated in arid and semi-arid zones with uncertain rainfall and poor soil. They provide a staple food in many parts of Africa and Asia, as gruel, porridge, and unleavened bread. Some millets have been cultivated in Europe and the USA.

Millet grain is often available in health food stores, although, unfortunately, exact identification is not given.

Nutritionally, millet grain follows the cereal pattern, although there are differences between species. The protein content varies between 8 and 12%. Millets have a good mineral content and high fibre. The grain is said to have a poor digestibility that is possibly linked to tannins in brown seed (a similar situation exists in sorghum). In some parts of India millet flour may be used to make chapattis, and there is some suggestion that these may have a lower glycaemic index than chapattis made from wheat flours.

Millet and sorghum do not contain gluten-forming proteins.

Table 18 Energy and nutrient content of millet and sorghum (per 100 g)

	Energy (kcal)	Protein (g)	Fat (g)	CHO^a (g)	NSP (g)	Calcium (mg)	Iron (mg)	Vitamin B$_1$ (mg)	Vitamin B$_2$ (mg)	Folate (µg)
Millet	378	11.0	4.2	72.9	N	8	3	0.42	0.29	–
Sorghum	339	11.3	3.3	74.9	N	28	4.4	0.24	0.14	–

^{a} CHO, carbohydrates; NSP, non-starch polysaccharides; N, no value available but likely to have significant amount; –, no value available.

Sorghum *Sorghum bicolor syn. S. vulgare*

Family Gramineae/Poaceae

Sorghum is an important human food in parts of Africa, South-east Asia, South America, and China. It may be consumed as porridge, roti or chapatti, tortilla, or other flat breads, and is used to make beer. Sorghum is gluten free.

Cereals

Buckwheat *Fagopyrum esculentum*

Family Polygonaceae

Cultivated in China, Japan, Russia, Poland, North America, Canada, and South Africa, buckwheat is not a cereal plant, but bears small black or grey seeds that resemble cereal grains. It has a high protein content (up to 11%) and the protein is high in lysine – the limiting amino acid in cereals. The flour does not contain gluten and therefore cannot be used on its own to make a leavened bread. It is usually eaten as porridge, pancakes, pasta, dumplings, and biscuits, often mixed with cereals. Buckwheat may be used with other ingredients, such as rice flour and potato flour, to make a composite gluten-free flour.

Table 19 Energy and some nutrients (per 100 g of buckwheat groats)

	Energy (kcal)	Protein (g)	Fat (g)	CHO[a] (g)	NSP (g)	Calcium (mg)	Iron (mg)	Vitamin B$_1$ (mg)	Vitamin B$_2$ (mg)	Folate (µg)
Buckwheat	364	8.1	1.5	84.9	2.1	12	4.9	0.28	0.07	–

[a] CHO, carbohydrates; NSP, non-starch polysaccharides; –, no value available.

Quinoa *Chenopodium quinoa*

Family Chenopodiaceae

This grain was grown in the high Andes and was a sacred food to the Incas. Today it is still used as a staple food in countries in South America, i.e. Argentina, Bolivia, Chile, Columbia, Equador, and Brazil. Small amounts are grown in the USA and UK.

The grain is unusually high in protein (up to 18%) and fat (4–9% – mainly unsaturated), and has less carbohydrate than the true cereals. Little is known about the vitamin content, although levels of B vitamins and carotene are said to be lower than in the cereals. However, it contains useful amounts of vitamin E and the minerals calcium and iron. The grain is sold in the whole, milled form and can be used in a similar way to rice or bulgar wheat. It is also available as flour, and used in breakfast cereals, bread, and soups. As it is gluten-free, quinoa is suitable for people with coeliac disease.

Table 20 Energy and some nutrients (per 100 g of quinoa grain)

	Energy (kcal)	Protein (g)	Fat (g)	CHO[a] (g)	NSP (g)	Calcium (mg)	Iron (mg)	Vitamin B$_1$ (mg)	Vitamin B$_2$ (mg)	Folate (µg)
Quinoa	374	13.1	5.8	68.9	N	60	9.3	0.20	0.40	–

[a] CHO, carbohydrates; NSP, non-starch polysaccharides; N, no value available but likely to have significant amount; –, no value available.

Cereals

Amaranth *Amaranthus species*

Family Amaranthaceae

Several *Amaranthus* species are grown as vegetables in various parts of the world (South-east Asia, Africa, and the Caribbean area), while *A. hypochondriacus*, *A. cruentus*, and *A. caudatus* have been cultivated as pseudo-cereal crops in Central America, South America, India, and Nepal. *A. caudatus* was the most important species grown by the Incas, Aztecs, and other pre-Colombian peoples – it is known as 'kiwicha'.

Amaranth seed and its products (e.g. cookies, breakfast foods, snacks, sweets) are now available in health food stores and supermarkets. Nutritionally, the grain is good, with a high level of protein containing the essential amino acid lysine (as explained previously, this is a deficiency in the major cereals).

Roman chamomile *Chamaemelum nobile syn. Anthemis nobilis;*
German chamomile *Matricaria recutita*

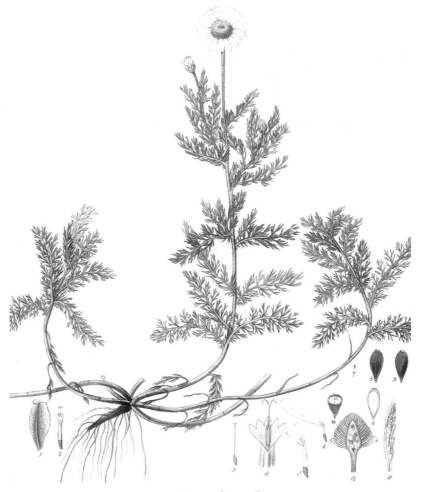

Roman chamomile.

Family Compositae/Asteraceae

ORIGIN AND CULTIVATION

The flower heads of both chamomile species are the source of herbal extracts.

- Roman (or English or garden lawn or sweet or true or double) chamomile: this is native to southern and western Europe and is cultivated in the UK, Belgium, the USA, Argentina, and other countries. It is the lawn chamomile.

- German (or Hungarian or single or wild) chamomile: this is native to Europe and northern and western Asia. It is extensively cultivated in Hungary, Romania, Bulgaria, the former Yugoslavia, Germany, Greece, and Egypt. German chamomile is produced in greater quantity than Roman chamomile.

PLANT DESCRIPTION

- Roman chamomile is a strongly fragrant (apple-like), much branched perennial with creeping stems 10–30 cm (12 in) long, and a height up to 0.3 m (1 ft). In the cultivated forms, the flower heads are normally double with mainly strap-shaped (ligulate) white florets, with possibly a few inner yellow disc florets. There is a conical solid receptacle covered with lance-shaped (lanceolate), membranous bracts.

- German chamomile is an annual growing up to 60 cm (24 in) in height. The flower heads have an outer single row of ligulate white florets and inner yellow disc florets. There is a conical hollow receptacle with no bracts.

Roman chamomile, German chamomile

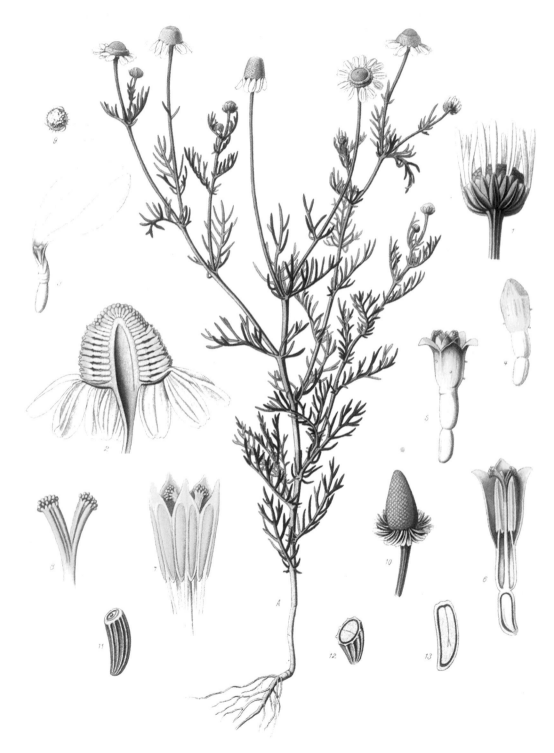

German chamomile.

Roman chamomile, German chamomile

CULINARY AND NUTRITIONAL VALUE

Blue essential oils are produced from the flower heads of both chamomiles by the processes of distillation or solvent extraction. These can be used as flavours in most major food categories: alcoholic beverages (bitters, vermouth, Benedictine liqueur), non-alcoholic beverages, frozen dairy desserts, confectionery, baked goods, jellies, and puddings.

CLAIMS AND FOLKLORE

Chamomile has been known since Roman times for its medical properties, and has been used in folk medicine to treat digestive and rheumatic disorders. Although information is available concerning the two chamomile types, preparations may contain both species.

Chamomile tea has a pleasant refreshing taste, and it has been suggested that there is more demand for it for tea than for medicinal purposes.

As regards medical claims:

- Roman chamomile is said to promote digestion, increase appetite, and be antiemetic, antispasmodic, and mildly sedative.

- German chamomile is the more often investigated of the two types and is used widely, certainly in Europe. Its essential oil has bactericidal and fungicidal properties. An infusion of flowers is said to have a marked hypnotic effect. Tea bags are used for insomnia, gout, sciatica, indigestion, and diarrhoea. It is claimed to have a particular place in children's ailments – colic, teething pains, and infantile convulsions.

Externally, infusions have been used to wash wounds and sores; the flowers have been employed as poultices; decoctions have been utilized as antispasmodic agents; and fresh or dried flowers in olive oil have been used to treat painful joints and swellings.

Extracts of both chamomile types have been included in pharmaceutical preparations, such as antiseptic ointments, and creams and gels for cracked nipples, sore gums, nappy rash, inflammation, and wound healing. In addition, extracts have been used in cosmetics, bath preparations, hair lighteners, shampoos, sunburn creams, and mouth washes. The oils have been utilized as fragrance components, and active ingredients in soaps, detergents, creams, lotions, and perfumes.

EVIDENCE

Roman and German chamomiles differ in the composition of their essential oils and other aspects of their chemistry, but certain compounds, such as some flavonoids, are common.

- The essential oil of Roman chamomile constitutes 0.4–1% of the flower head and contains a number of constituents, including aliphatic esters of angelic and tiglic acids. In addition to the essential oil, the flower head contains sesquiterpene lactones, flavonoids, and coumarins.

- German chamomile produces up to 2% essential oil, which contains alpha-bisabolol (about 50%), azulenes, and other constituents. As with Roman chamomile, the flower head holds a variety of chemical substances besides the essential oil.

A large number of experiments, involving both humans and animals, have been carried out on the efficacy of the chamomiles, particularly the German type. There is widespread support for many of the herbal uses (e.g. anti-inflammatory and antispasmodic activities).

Chamomile may be taken as a tea, but also as a liquid extract (with alcohol). The low water solubility of the essential oil means that a tea only contains about 10–15% of the oil in the plant.

The excessive use of the chamomiles during pregnancy and lactation should be avoided, although on the whole they are regarded as safe. Nevertheless, persons allergic to ragwort, asters, chrysanthemums, and other members of the Compositae/Asteraceae family should be cautious about drinking infusions. German, but not Roman chamomile is supported in Germany.

Chickweed *Stellaria media*

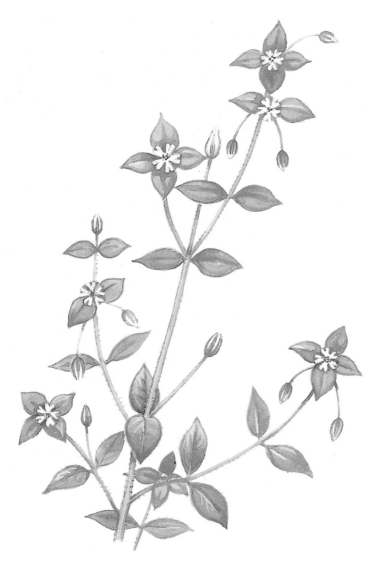

Family Caryophyllaceae

ORIGIN AND CULTIVATION
Chickweed is found in cultivated and waste places throughout Europe and northern Asia. It has been carried as a weed to all other temperate regions of the world.

PLANT DESCRIPTION
It is an annual with straggling stems 10–40 cm (16 in) long, and ovate, pointed leaves. Star-like white flowers are produced.

The whole plant is employed in herbal medicine.

CULINARY AND NUTRITIONAL VALUE
Chickweed has been included in salads, cooked as a vegetable, and given as food to animals. It contains vitamin C (150–375 mg per 100 g) and other vitamins.

CLAIMS AND FOLKLORE
In herbal medicine, chickweed is regarded as having cooling and demulcent properties, and so has been included in ointments and poultices to treat various skin disorders (rashes, sores, boils, and other ailments). It has been used internally for chest ailments, although its external use, as so far described, has been more important.

EVIDENCE
Chemical analysis has identified coumarins, glycosides, flavonoids, saponins, and some other substances. Although chickweed has been used for centuries, there seems to be no experimental evidence to support its claimed therapeutic value.

It should not be used during pregnancy, and it has been stated that too much chickweed may cause diarrhoea or nitrate poisoning.

Coenzyme Q_{10} (or ubiquinone Q_{10})

ORIGIN

Coenzyme Q_{10} was discovered in 1957 and is found in every cell of the human body. It is located in the subcellular structures known as 'mitochondria', and is a substance essential for the production of energy. Cells with a large energy requirement (e.g. heart, muscles, liver) contain high numbers of mitochondria.

We can obtain Q_{10} from food (e.g. various meats, eggs, fatty fish, wholemeal products, nuts, many vegetables), but it is also made within the body, namely in the liver, and this internal production is greater than that obtained from food. The daily intake of Q_{10} from food is in the region of 5–15 mg.

It is stated that the amount of Q_{10} in the body can be reduced through various illnesses or ageing; therefore, as Q_{10} is essential for energy production, a dietary supplement of the substance has sometimes been recommended. Q_{10} supplements are produced synthetically.

CULINARY AND NUTRITIONAL VALUE

None.

CLAIMS AND FOLKLORE

As Q_{10} is a recently discovered substance, there is no established folklore, such as with many herbal medicines and some other supplements. Nevertheless, it is taken as a food supplement by many – some 10 million Japanese people are said to use it!

Because of the essential part Q_{10} plays in the production of energy, claims for the therapeutic value of the substance are often based on this function. During ageing, as previously stated, the amount of Q_{10} drops, so that a supplement might be claimed to improve the energy of the elderly. People suffering from various heart diseases have low concentrations of Q_{10} in the heart muscle. Some clinical studies have alleged that supplementation with Q_{10} has improved the situation. Other conditions that have supposedly been improved with Q_{10} dosage include diseases causing loose teeth; it is also said to promote endurance in athletes.

Q_{10} is an antioxidant (see Introduction).

EVIDENCE

There is considerable scientific interest in Q_{10} – occasional international meetings take place, but these are not concerned entirely with the therapeutic value of the substance. A number of animal and human trials have been carried out into the therapeutic value of Q_{10} and the results are interesting, but more research is required. For example, the recommended daily allowance is 10–30 mg, although when treating illnesses 100–300 g may be used. Clearly, more exact information about dosage would be desirable. Experiments have shown that Q_{10} is best absorbed by the body if taken dissolved in soya oil in soft capsules; granulated and tablet preparations are not nearly so effective.

It seems well accepted that Q_{10} acts as an antioxidant but whether its claimed therapeutic value is related to this function or to the part it plays in the energy chain is not clear. Also well accepted is the non-toxic nature of Q_{10} – even at high doses.

Certain prescription drugs (e.g. cholesterol lowering, beta-blockers, sulphonylureas for diabetes) can inhibit Q_{10} production in the body – a possible reason for supplementation.

Coltsfoot *Tussilago farfara*

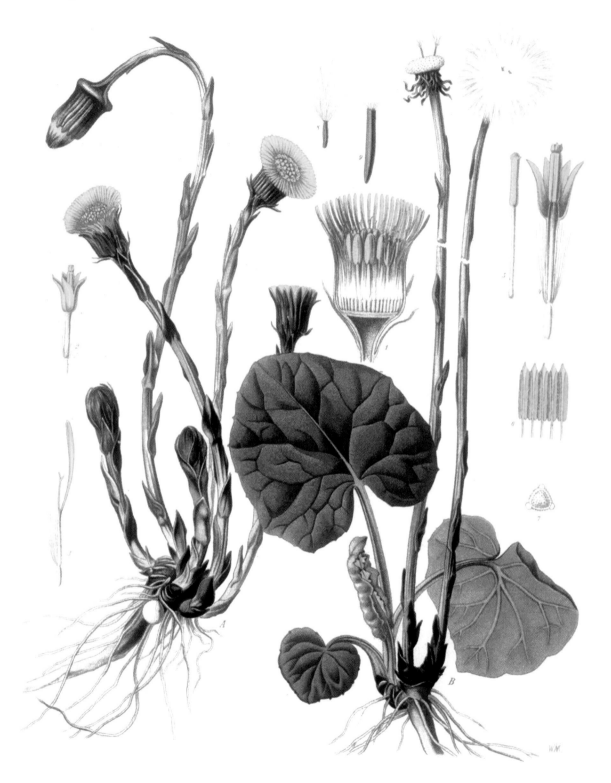

Coltsfoot

Family Compositae/Asteraceae

ORIGIN AND CULTIVATION
Coltsfoot is native to Europe, but it also grows widely throughout other countries, including the USA, Canada, and China. The herb is collected from wild plants in the Balkans, eastern Europe, and Italy. It has been part of Chinese folk medicine for centuries.

PLANT DESCRIPTION
The plant is a low growing perennial, which, first of all in the spring (February–April), produces a flowering stem up to 30 cm (12 in) high, terminated by a flower head (up to 2 cm in diameter) consisting of golden-yellow, narrow, strap-shaped florets. After the flower dies back, the leaves appear (May–June). These are hoof shaped, about 10 cm (3 in) in diameter, with a green upper surface and a lower surface covered with white hairs.

NUTRITIONAL AND CULINARY VALUE
Coltsfoot extracts are sometimes used as flavourings for candies and confectionery.

CLAIMS AND FOLKLORE
Extracts of buds, flowers, and leaves have long been used in traditional medicine (including Chinese) for the treatment of dry cough, throat irritation, bronchitis, and other respiratory diseases. It has been available in tablets, liquid medicines, and teas (often mixed with other herbs).

A smoking mixture of coltsfoot and other herbs has been available for the management of coughs and wheezes.

EVIDENCE
Coltsfoot contains a number of different chemical substances, including tannins, mucilage (about 8%), alkaloids, carotenoids, and flavonoids. Probably the composition of leaves and flowers is different.

As stated, the herb has long been used to soothe sore throats. This therapeutic value is normally related to the mucilage. If this is the case, it is strange that coltsfoot is included in smoking mixtures to ease coughs, because burning will destroy the mucilage and, in addition, smoke will irritate the throat.

A number of animal experiments have suggested other possible activities of coltsfoot. As in ginkgo, it has been claimed that coltsfoot possesses an inhibitor of the platelet-activating factor concerned with chronic asthma and other inflammatory diseases. It has also been suggested that the mucilage is anti-inflammatory and possibly acts as an immunostimulant. The flavonoids present might have anti-inflammatory and antispasmodic properties.

Care must be taken with the quantity of coltsfoot used because of the presence of alkaloids (pyrrolizidine), which are possibly carcinogenic. Indeed, the use of coltsfoot is not recommended by some authorities. In Germany there is strict control of coltsfoot products. They should not be used during pregnancy and lactation.

Comfrey, knitbone *Symphytum officinale*

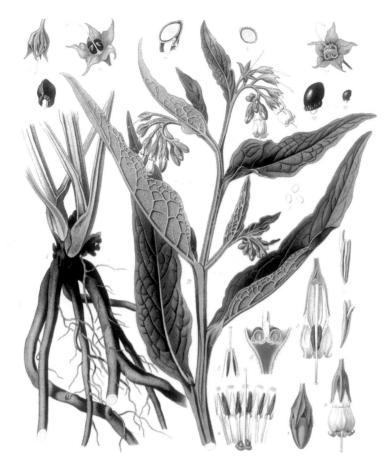

Family Boraginaceae

ORIGIN AND CULTIVATION

Comfrey grows in moist grasslands and on riverbanks in Europe, western Asia, North America, and Australia. Russian comfrey, grown as a fodder crop for cattle, evolved as a hybrid between *Symphytum officinale* and prickly comfrey (*S. asperum*).

PLANT DESCRIPTION

Comfrey grows to a height of 60–100 cm (3 ft), and has a thick brown rootstock (rhizome) and mucilaginous roots. The plant is a bristly-haired perennial with large, oval, lanceolate leaves. Its flowers are funnel shaped and white to purple.

The parts used in herbal medicine are the rhizome, root, and leaf.

CULINARY AND NUTRITIONAL VALUE

The young leaves have been used as a vegetable, but this practice is discouraged because of the presence of toxic alkaloids (pyrrolizidine).

CLAIMS AND FOLKLORE

Comfrey has been used in herbal medicine for centuries – it was known to Dioscorides in the first century. The herb has been employed in the treatment of chronic bronchial disease, gastric and duodenal ulcers, colitis, rheumatism (leaf tea only), and irritable bowel syndrome. Externally, it has been applied to broken bones (hence one of its names), bruises, sprains, fractures, psoriasis, eczema, and other skin conditions.

EVIDENCE

Of the various chemical substances present in comfrey, allantoin (0.75–2.55%) is said to possess cell-proliferating properties that could assist in tissue healing.

Animal studies have indicated that rosmarinic acid has anti-inflammatory activity.

Much attention has been paid to the alkaloids (pyrrolizidine) (0.3%) in the roots and leaves. These alkaloids are toxic to the liver and, in a number of countries, tablets, capsules, and other products containing comfrey for internal use have been withdrawn from sale. However, comfrey tea seems to be tolerated, possibly because of the low alkaloid concentration.

There is apparently little or no objection to the use of comfrey in ointments, balms, and other products for the external treatment of the unbroken skin, and as long as the treatment is not prolonged. In Germany, comfrey products are applied externally to bruises and sprains, but there is a limit to the pyrrolizidine alkaloids contained in the product. Possibly mucilage in comfrey helps soften the skin.

Cramp bark, guelder rose *Viburnum opulus;*
black haw bark *V. prunifolium*

Family Caprifoliaceae

ORIGIN AND CULTIVATION
Cramp bark is found in hedgerows and woods in Europe, parts of Asia, and the USA. Black haw grows in parts of North America.

PLANT DESCRIPTION
- *Viburnum opulus*: this is a deciduous shrub with 3–5-lobed leaves 4–7 cm (3 in) broad, growing to a height of 4 m (13 ft).

The small white flowers (except the outer ones, which may become 2 cm ($\frac{4}{5}$ in) wide) are in flat clusters giving rise to globular blackish red fruits.

- *V. prunifolium*: this is a deciduous shrub or small tree 5–9 m (30 ft) high. The arrangement of flowers is as in *V. opulus*, and the fruits are blue–black.

The parts used, in both species, are the stem and root barks.

CULINARY AND NUTRITIONAL VALUE
In the USA, fruits of *V. prunifolium* have been used for preserves since colonial times; however, it is stated that they (and those of *V. opulus*) are poisonous when raw but edible when cooked. Extracts have been used as flavour ingredients in alcoholic and non-alcoholic beverages.

CLAIMS AND FOLKLORE
Extracts of both species have been used internally as an antispasmodic, a sedative, and for nervous constipation, and externally for muscular cramp. The drug has been particularly employed for dealing with painful menstruation and other gynaecological problems, by the American Indians, amongst others.

EVIDENCE
Both species contain several active constituents, including the coumarin scopoletin, hydroquinones, various acids, and tannins. *V. prunifolium* also contains salicin; therefore, people allergic to aspirin should not use the herbal extract.

Some experimental studies support the action of these herbal extracts as uterine antispasmodics *in vitro*.

Cranberry, American cranberry

Vaccinium oxycoccus, V. macrocarpon

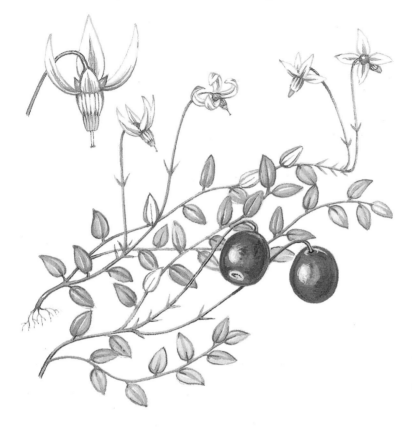

Family Ericaceae

ORIGIN AND CULTIVATION

Cranberry (*Vaccinium oxycoccus*) is a native of northern Europe, northern Asia, and North America, and is found growing in peat bogs. Some fruits are gathered in the wild and there has been small-scale cultivation. However, as regards commercial cultivation, it has been replaced by the American cranberry (*V. macrocarpon*), which is grown in some parts of the USA, Canada, and the UK.

PLANT DESCRIPTION

V. oxycoccus is a small, prostrate plant with thin stems and oblong or elliptical leaves, 4–10 mm ($\frac{2}{5}$ in) long. The flowers are borne singly or in pairs, with dark pink petals, 5–6 mm ($\frac{1}{4}$ in) long. Fruits are red, rounded, or oval, 4–6 mm ($\frac{1}{4}$ in) across. *V. macrocarpon* is a larger version of the previous species, with fruits 12–20 mm ($\frac{4}{5}$ in) across.

CULINARY AND NUTRITIONAL VALUE

The fruit is used in cranberry jelly and sauce – traditional additions to venison and turkey – and there is now a significant market in cranberry juice. The fruit contains about 4% sugars (more glucose than fructose) and 13 mg per 100 g vitamin C with high levels of several acids (e.g. citric, malic, quinic, benzoic).

CLAIMS AND FOLKLORE

Cranberries (fruits) have been used in eastern Europe, in their folklore role, for the treatment of cancers and to reduce fever.

Probably the most interesting claim, made in the mid-1800s in Germany, was that the urinary excretion of hippuric acid increased after the ingestion of cranberries. It was believed that cranberries (and prunes and plums) contained benzoic acid or some other compounds that the body metabolized and excreted as hippuric acid, which was said to counteract bacterial infection.

EVIDENCE

Possibly, not a great deal of scientific evidence is available; nevertheless, interest in its medical use still persists. The ingestion of cranberry leads to an increased urine acidity, which might relieve urinary tract infection and reduce the incidence of some kinds of kidney stones. Recent studies have suggested that it is not acidity that inhibits bacterial growth but a chemical mechanism that prevents bacteria from adhering to the lining of the urinary tract. Clearly, more experimental work is required.

An interesting suggestion is that cranberry be used as a urinary deodorant in incontinent patients. It has been suggested that ingestion of the juice would increase the acidity of urine, and thus retard the bacterial degradation which normally leads to the pungent ammonia odour.

Cranberry is generally non-toxic. It is reasonable to suggest that cranberry products could well be a useful adjunct to treatment for urinary infections.

Dairy products

Dairy products are usually regarded as animal milks and the products made from them. In the UK 'milk' usually means cow's milk, but goat's and sheep's milk are becoming increasingly available. Yoghurt and cheese may be made from any of these milks.

Milk and dairy products became important sources of energy, protein, and other nutrients in programmes to improve nutrition both before and during the Second World War. They therefore came to be seen as 'good' foods. In affluent societies, however, the fatty acid composition of the milk (relatively saturated), and the suggestion that people may be sensitive either to the protein or the lactose in animal milks, has led to something of a fall from grace.

The nutritional characteristics of mammalian milks are shown in Table 21. The nutritional composition of different species' milk varies, leading to the comment that each is designed by nature to feed the specific animal and that that is what it should be used for. In any case, most would agree that human milk is the best for the human infant, although, for those who cannot be fed in this way, suitable 'humanized' formulae are invaluable. Generally, milks supply useful amounts of protein, fat, and carbohydrate – the latter in the form of lactose. They are also important sources of calcium in the diet, cow's milk containing less than sheep's milk but more than goat's.

The fat in cow's milk is relatively saturated, because fermentation of food in the rumen of the animal leads to saturation of the fatty acids in the animal feedstuff. Milks with varying levels of fat are therefore now produced, as shown in Table 22, and consumption of these has now overtaken consumption of whole milk. Other milk products you may find include evaporated milk, where the nutrients are concentrated due to loss of water, and condensed milk, in which the milk is concentrated and has sugar added. The fat separated from the milk is sold as cream. Single cream contains about 18% fat (200 kcal per

Table 21 Composition of commonly consumed animal milks (per 100 g)

Constituent	Cow	Goat	Sheep	Human (mature)
Water (g)	87.9	88.9	83.0	88.2
Energy (kcal)	66	60	95	69
Energy (kJ)	276	253	396	289
Protein (g)	3.1	3.2	5.4	1.0
Fat (g)	3.9	3.5	6.0	4.1
Lactose (g)	4.6	4.4	5.1	7.2
Calcium (mg)	115	100	170	34

100 g), whipping cream 39% (375 kcal), and double cream about 48% fat (450 kcal).

INTOLERANCE TO COW'S MILK

There are two potential problems, the first relating to the proteins in the milk (cow's milk protein intolerance) and the second relating to the lactose in milk (lactose intolerance).

Protein intolerance

Allergy or intolerance to cow's milk protein usually develops in early infancy when the baby is exposed to cow's milk in infant formulae or as milk. It rarely appears after the age of 12 months, and 90% of children recover by the age of three. It causes gastrointestinal symptoms such as vomiting and diarrhoea, irritability, and failure to thrive (i.e. poor growth and weight gain). True cow's milk protein allergy, where an immunological basis can be found, is often associated with a family history of allergy, with symptoms such as eczema, asthma, and rhinitis (runny nose). Treatment of cow's milk protein allergy, or cow's milk protein intolerance is the same: removal of all cow's milk and products made from it from the diet. This should not be attempted in infancy or childhood without advice from a registered dietitian, as a suitable nutri-

Table 22 Energy and nutrient content of milk products (per 100 g)

Constituent	Semi-skimmed[a]	Skimmed	Dried skimmed	Evaporated whole[b]	Condensed whole[b]
Water (g)	89.9	91.1	3.0	69.1	25.9
Energy (kcal)	46	33	350	151	333
Energy (kJ)	195	140	1491	664	1406
Protein (g)	3.3	3.3	36.1	8.4	8.5
Fat (g)	1.6	0.1	1.0	9.4	10.1
Lactose (g)	4.7	5.0	52.9	8.5	12.3
Calcium (mg)	120	120	1280	290	290

[a]So-called 2% milk in US and Europe.
[b]Both of these milks may also be made from skimmed milk and will then have a lower fat content.

Dairy products

tionally complete substitute formula will be required. Many children who are allergic to cow's milk protein are also allergic to soya milks and therefore cannot take these or products made from them. The best replacement formulae for children are usually those where the protein has been hydrolysed so that the body does not recognize the proteins.

In older children and adults who may be intolerant to cow's milk protein, goat's or sheep's milk may be an alternative. However some people may not tolerate these milks either, and goat's milk is low in folates compared with cow's milk. There have also been concerns about microbial contamination with these milks, so care should be taken to ensure that only pasteurized products are used. Plant milks may provide an alternative to animal milks in these cases.

Lactose intolerance

This results from an inability to digest the disaccharide, lactose, which is the sugar present in animal milks, including those of sheep, goats, and humans. There is an extremely rare condition where babies are born with an inability to digest lactose and therefore cannot even take breast milk. Sometimes lactose intolerance may occur after gastroenteritis or operations on the gut, but this is usually temporary; in both cases dietetic advice will be needed.

However, lactose intolerance is very common in some racial groups because there is a reduction in lactase, the enzyme that breaks down lactose in the food, in the gut after infancy. People with this type of lactose intolerance may be able to tolerate small amounts of milk, but will develop symptoms such as diarrhoea and bloating if they drink large amounts. They also need to be aware that it may be necessary to avoid medicines in which lactose is used as the main part of a tablet carrying a drug.

Unlike cow's milk protein intolerance, lactose intolerance does not require the removal of dairy products such as cheese and yoghurt from the diet, as most of the lactose is converted to lactic acid during fermentation in yoghurt, or removed in the cheese-making process. Yoghurts containing probiotic bacteria (see p. 125) seem to be particularly beneficial in people with lactose intolerance, and it is thought that the probiotic bacteria may produce a lactase, which helps to digest the lactose in the milk.

Lactose-free milks

These are milks that have had a lactase enzyme added to them so that the lactose has been broken down to the simple sugars (glucose and galactose) that make it up. These milks are, therefore, suitable for older children and adults who cannot tolerate lactose – but not for infants who need a nutritionally complete formula free of lactose.

Lactase is also available in liquid or tablet form. This can be added to ordinary milk, and left for several hours to allow the lactose to be broken down.

PLANT MILKS

A variety of plant 'milks' are available. The most commonly used is soya milk (see p. 146), but cereal milks and nut milks are also available. These are free of cow's milk protein and lactose, and the nutrient content of plant milks is shown in Table 23. Some people have allergic reactions to the proteins in soya or nuts, so care should be taken with these.

YOGHURT

Yoghurt is a fermented milk product. Fermentation of milk with *Lactobacillus* species leads to the production of lactic acid from the lactose, and the acidification of the milk prevents the growth of pathogenic bacteria – thus stabilizing the milk. Yoghurt originated in south-east Europe and Turkey, where milk is fermented with *Lactobacillus bulgaricus* to form a soft curd. Yoghurts are made from cow's or

Table 23 Nutrient composition of plant 'milks' compared to semi-skimmed cow's milk (per 100 g)

Constituent	Semi-skimmed cow's milk	Soya 'milk'	Oat 'milk'	Rice 'milk'	Almond 'milk'	Hazelnut 'milk'
Energy (kcal)	46	47	50	50	53	40
Energy (kJ)	195	196	209	209	222	167
Protein (g)	3.3	3.6	1.8	0.4	1	0.6
Fat (g)	1.6	2.5	0.7	0.8	2.6	2.1
Carbohydrate (g)	4.7	2.6	9.5	10.4	6.5	4.6
Calcium (mg)	120	91[a]	8[b]	120[c]	12[b]	7[b]

[a] Calcium enriched (in the un-enriched product, the calcium content is about 13 mg per 100 g).
[b] Un-enriched; calculated by dilution of calcium content of oats or nuts using protein content to set proportions. Some varieties may be fortified – see labels.
[c] Calcium enriched.

Dairy products

goat's milk (soya milk yoghurts are also now being made) and may be produced from whole, semi-skimmed, or skimmed milk. They provide the same range of nutrients as the milk from which they are produced, without the lactose. Some yoghurts are therefore quite high in fat, others are low in fat. Some have sugar added, and some may also have fruit or fruit purées or other flavours added.

Yoghurt has a much reduced lactose content as the sugar is fermented to lactic acid during manufacture.

'Bio-' or 'live' yoghurts contain live cultures of bacteria. Some yoghurts are now made with specific strains of *Lactobacillus* or *Bifidobacter*, which have specific 'probiotic' effects (see p. 125).

Damiana *Turnera diffusa var. aphrodisiaca syn. T. aphrodisiaca*

Family Turneraceae

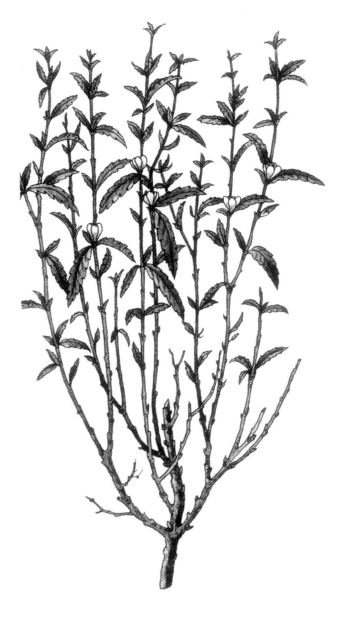

ORIGIN AND CULTIVATION
Damiana grows in dry, sandy, and rocky places in southern North America, Central America, northern South America, and Namibia.

PLANT DESCRIPTION
The plant is an aromatic, shrubby perennial with toothed leaves, up to 2.5 cm (1 in) in length. Its flowers are yellow to orange in colour and give rise to aromatic fruits about 2 cm ($\frac{4}{5}$ in) across. The plant grows to a height of about 1 m (3 ft).

The leaves are the source of the herbal drug.

CULINARY AND NUTRITIONAL VALUE
It has been included as an ingredient of liqueurs produced in Mexico.

CLAIMS AND FOLKLORE
Damiana was used by the Maya people of Central America to treat giddiness and loss of balance. In most recent times it has been promoted as an aphrodisiac. Damiana has also been used as a tonic, laxative, and urinary antiseptic, and as an antidepressant.

EVIDENCE
Among the chemical compounds identified in damiana are an essential oil (containing at least 20 components) responsible for the characteristic odour and taste, tannins, and glycosides.

There is no experimental work to support the use of damiana as an aphrodisiac. Because of the presence of glycosides, care should be observed in using the drug, including in pregnancy and lactation. It is not recommended in Germany.

Dandelion *Taraxacum officinale*

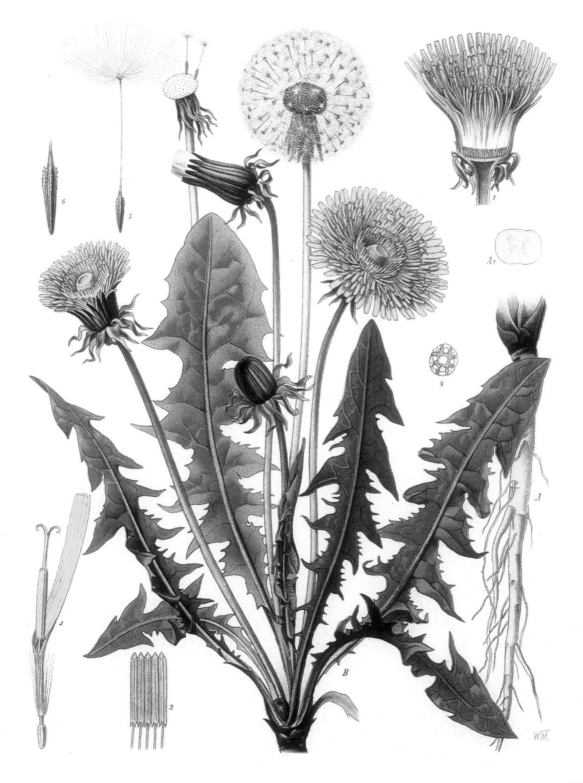

Dandelion

Family Compositae/Asteraceae

ORIGIN AND CULTIVATION

Dandelion is found in the temperate areas of Europe and Asia, and has spread to many other parts of the world. Forms, selected for large leaves to be used in salads, may well still be cultivated in gardens in France.

PLANT DESCRIPTION

It is a perennial, with a basal rosette of leaves dissected to varying degrees. The flower stalk, which may attain a height of 50 cm (20 in), carries a flower head 2–6 cm (2 in) across, consisting of strap-shaped yellow florets that give rise to the well known parachute-like fruits. There is a strong taproot.

CULINARY AND NUTRITIONAL VALUE

The young leaves, blanched or soaked in water to remove bitterness, are included in salads. They have a high content of carotenoids (greater than carrots) that are precursors to vitamin A. There is also a large amount of potassium (297 mg per 100 g) in the leaf.

Its leaves and roots can be used to flavour herbal beers and soft drinks (e.g. dandelion and burdock). From the root is made a caffeine-free coffee, and from the flowers, a wine. The root contains about 25% inulin, which could be employed to produce a high-fructose syrup.

CLAIMS AND FOLKLORE

Analyses of dandelion have indicated a wide range of chemical substances, including terpenoids and sesquiterpene lactones.

The plant has been used in herbal medicine for a very long time, both in Europe and the East. Its root has been employed as a diuretic (a common name is 'wet-the-bed', in French *pissenlit*), tonic, laxative, and appetite stimulant, and to stimulate bile flow. The root and leaves have been used to treat heartburn, flatulence, bruises, chronic rheumatism, gout, and skin problems. The leaves, too, can act as a powerful diuretic, with the added advantage that the high percentage of potassium means that some is retained in the body, although there is a considerable loss in urine.

EVIDENCE

Although dandelion has a long history in herbal medicine, there seems to have been relatively little investigation into its efficacy. However, animal studies have certainly confirmed its powerful diuretic action. It should not be used by those with blocked bile ducts. Approval is given to the drug in Germany.

Deadly nightshade *Atropa belladonna*

Family Solanaceae

ORIGIN AND CULTIVATION

Deadly nightshade is found growing in northern, central, and southern Europe, Asia Minor, and North Africa. It is cultivated world-wide, including in the USA, UK, China, and India. The plant grows on wasteland and wooded hills; it seems to flourish best on calcareous soils and in the shade.

PLANT DESCRIPTION

This perennial herb grows to a height of 1.0–1.5 m (5 ft), has fleshy roots, and an erect branched stem with ovate leaves up to 20 cm (8 in) long. The purple, bell-shaped flowers give rise to shiny black berries, about the size of small cherries.

The parts used are the roots, leaves, and berries.

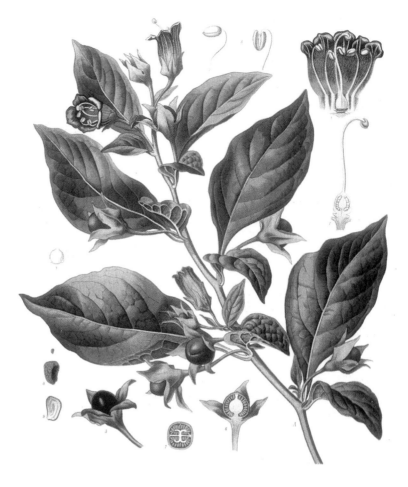

NUTRITIONAL AND CULINARY VALUE

None.

CLAIMS AND FOLKLORE

The plant has a long usage in practice and folklore. It was included in witches' brew to simulate the feeling of flying and, in the Middle Ages, Italian women used the berry juice to enlarge the pupil to give the eye a glistening appearance.

Like all plants, deadly nightshade contains a variety of chemical substances, but the action of its extracts is normally related to alkaloids (tropane): hyoscyamine, scopolamine, and atropine. These alkaloids are included in prescription medicines, and have an antispasmodic effect on the digestive system, bladder, and urethra. They also reduce anxiety or nervous tension and relieve insomnia. In eye examinations, the alkaloids will dilate the pupil.

As regards over-the-counter medicines, belladonna is included in liniments, in homeopathic preparations for acne, boils, and sunburn, and in medicines for the topical treatment of rheumatism, sciatica, and similar complaints.

EVIDENCE

As far as can be discovered, there is no experimental evidence to support the use of belladonna in homeopathic medicine. The inclusion of the drug in prescribed medicines seems to be well supported, as is its use in topical preparations available over the counter.

However, it should be made clear that all parts of deadly nightshade are very poisonous and should not be ingested. The toxicity effects are quite startling. Adulteration of other herb roots with those of deadly nightshade has led to unpleasant situations. It has been suggested that deadly nightshade material should not be brought into contact with broken skin, and its use is not advisable during pregnancy and lactation. It is not supported in Germany.

Devil's claw *Harpagophytum procumbens*

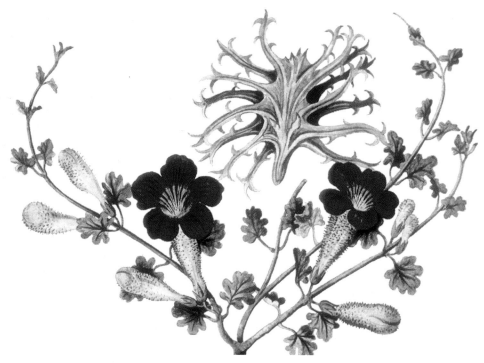

Family Pedaliaceae

ORIGIN AND CULTIVATION

Devil's claw grows wild in southern Africa, particularly in the Kalahari desert and Namibia, and Madagascar. It is a hazard to animals that pick up the thorny fruits in their coats. It is said that it was introduced to Western medicine by G.H. Mehnert, a South African farmer who observed local people using decoctions of the dried tuber to treat various ailments, e.g. rheumatism.

The plant is now cultivated to some extent in southern Africa, for export of the dried tuber to Europe.

PLANT DESCRIPTION

H. procumbens is a trailing perennial up to 1.5 m (5 ft) in length, with tubers possibly 20 cm (8 in) long and 6 cm (2 in) thick, producing many aerial stems bearing round to ovate toothed or pinnately lobed leaves, about 7 cm (3 in) long, with white hairy undersides. The colourful flowers are up to 6 cm (2 in) long, solitary, red to purple, trumped shaped, and appear in the spring. These flowers give rise to dehiscent capsules (fruits), up to 7 cm (3 in) in length and armed with barbed thorns 2.5 cm (1 in) long, said to be used as mouse traps in Madagascar!

CULINARY AND NUTRITIONAL VALUE

None.

CLAIMS AND FOLKLORE

In traditional medicine in Africa, and since the early twentieth century in Europe, extracts of the dried tuber have been used to treat rheumatism, arthritis, digestive problems, headache, allergies, lumbago, neuralgia, and other conditions, including cancer.

As a health food it is found in herb teas, tablets, capsules, and extracts (e.g. tinctures), and is primarily taken as a relief for arthritic symptoms.

EVIDENCE

Among the various chemicals present in devil's claw, harpagide and harpagoside (iridoid glycosides) are regarded as the active anti-inflammatory principles effective in the use of the drug for arthritic symptoms. Some investigations with animals, and humans, have been carried out into the efficacy of devil's claw and the results are promising. More human studies are required.

The drug should not be given to patients with gastric or duodenal ulcers, and should not be used during pregnancy and lactation. It is supported in Germany.

Dried fruits

Fresh fruit is an essential part of a healthy diet, but health food shops usually only sell dried fruits. The nutritional content of these depends to a large extent on the composition of the fresh fruit, which is described below. Fruits are a major source of vitamin C (citrus 40–80 mg per 100 g; blackcurrant 70–190 mg per 100 g). Other vitamins (e.g. E, B_1, B_2, and folate) are also present, but not in such large quantities. Various fruits (e.g. mango, papaya, and apricot) are good sources of the orange–red pigments, carotenes, some of which are precursors of vitamin A. Fruits also provide useful amounts of minerals, such as calcium and iron, with usually high amounts of potassium (fresh dates 400 mg per 100 g; apricots 300 mg per 100 g). Flavour and aroma are important in a diet. Sweetness is related to the sugars present (sucrose, glucose, fructose), and organic acids (citric and malic) are other flavour components. Numerous volatile compounds (e.g. esters, alcohols, and aldehydes) are also involved in flavour and aroma. Colour, too, is important in diet, and in fruits there are the orange–red carotenes and the red and purple anthocyanins. Fruits are a source of fibre (soluble and insoluble). Protein and fat are present in small quantities.

The drying of materials has been an important method of food preservation since time immemorial. A low content of water inhibits or prevents the growth of spoilage microorganisms.

PROCESSING

Fruit can be dried either by the sun or mechanical dehydrators. In some cases, drying is preceded by sulphuring, i.e. treatment with burning sulphur or gaseous sulphur dioxide. The amount of sulphur dioxide must be controlled, and is subject to regulations that vary from country to country. One of the objects of sulphuring is to preserve the colour of dried fruits and to prevent enzymatic browning. It has also been claimed that it reduces the destruction of carotene and vitamin C (see under nutritional value). The moisture content of dried fruits varies from species to species, e.g. apricot, 15–20%; peaches, less than 4%; pears, 15–25%; apple, 20%; dates, 15%; figs, 16%; and pineapple, 10%.

Many different types of fruits are dried. These include, in addition to those above, bananas, grapes (currants, raisins, sultanas), plums (prunes), and others.

CULINARY AND NUTRITIONAL VALUE

Dried fruits can be eaten alone, or used in baking, various recipes, desserts, and confections. They provide flavour and, in some cases, such as cakes, no additional water.

Drying concentrates those nutrients that are not heat or light labile. Vitamin C is the main casualty, often being reduced to a mere trace, but other vitamins are not overaffected. Concentration affects the important constituents of dried fruit, e.g. 10% total sugars in fresh apple increase to about 60% in dried apple; in dried pineapple they are 70%, up from 10%. This will control the amount of energy available, e.g. from fresh to dried pineapple there is an increase from 40 to 280 kcal per 100 g; in figs an increase from 40 to 230 kcal. Minerals, too, will be concentrated; e.g. in apricots, potassium increases from about 270 to 1900 mg per 100 g. Dietary fibre is also concentrated on drying, e.g. in figs, from 2 to 12% and, in pineapple, from 1 to 9%.

ANTINUTRITIONAL SUBSTANCES

Dried fruits may become infected with fungal moulds, often species of *Aspergillus* and *Penicillium*. These moulds can produce chemical substances known as mycotoxins, which may be carcinogenic. The mycotoxin aflatoxin may be found in dried figs and fig products, and dates. Ochratoxin can be a particular problem in raisins, currants, and sultanas, but has also been found in dried figs, dates, and apricots. Patulin can be a problem in fruit juice and jam, particularly apple juice.

Official regulations in various countries determine the acceptable upper limits for these mycotoxins.

FRUIT JUICES

Extracted fruit juice may be modified in various ways, e.g. by sweetening or concentrating. Generally speaking, juices contain the same range and almost the same concentrations of nutrients as fruits, except dietary fibre, which is low, and vitamin C, which varies according to packaging and length of storage. The sugars in fruit juice are absorbed more rapidly than those in the whole fruit, thus giving a higher glycaemic response (see p. xv).

Drosera, sundew *Drosera rotundifolia*

Family Droseraceae

ORIGIN AND CULTIVATION

Drosera rotundifolia is found in bogs and wet ground throughout temperate Europe, Japan, and North America. Two other species – *D. longifolia* and *D. anglica* – may also be utilized. *D. madagascariensis* is exported from Madagascar. *Drosera* material is normally taken from wild stock, and there are fears of serious depletion. Consequently, some countries employ restrictions. In Finland there is research into the cultivation of the plant.

PLANT DESCRIPTION

The plant is a perennial, with a rosette of rounded leaves covered with red sticky tentacles or hairs for trapping insects. White flowers, borne on aerial stems up to 10–15 cm (6 in) in height, give rise to capsular fruits.

The whole plant is used in herbal medicine.

CULINARY AND NUTRITIONAL VALUE

Sundew liqueur was popular in Britain, France, and Germany during the seventeenth century.

CLAIMS AND FOLKLORE

Extracts of the plant are said to have antispasmodic, demulcent, and expectorant properties, and have been used to treat asthma, bronchitis, gastritis, whooping cough, and some other conditions.

EVIDENCE

Among other chemical substances, drosera contains naphthoquinones (e.g. plumbagin), which are supposed to be the active constituents. Animal experiments support some of the properties attributed to drosera, e.g. an antispasmodic action, and its extracts show some antimicrobial properties. Drosera is not recommended for use during pregnancy and lactation. It is supported in Germany.

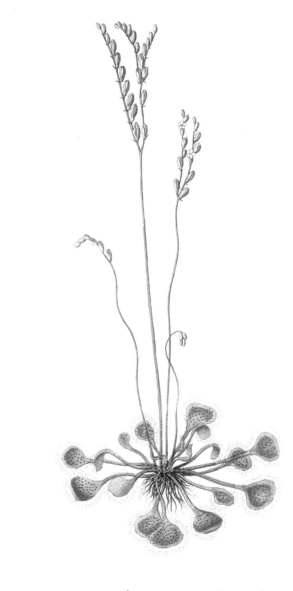

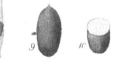

Echinacea, coneflower

Echinacea purpurea, E. angustifolia, E. pallida

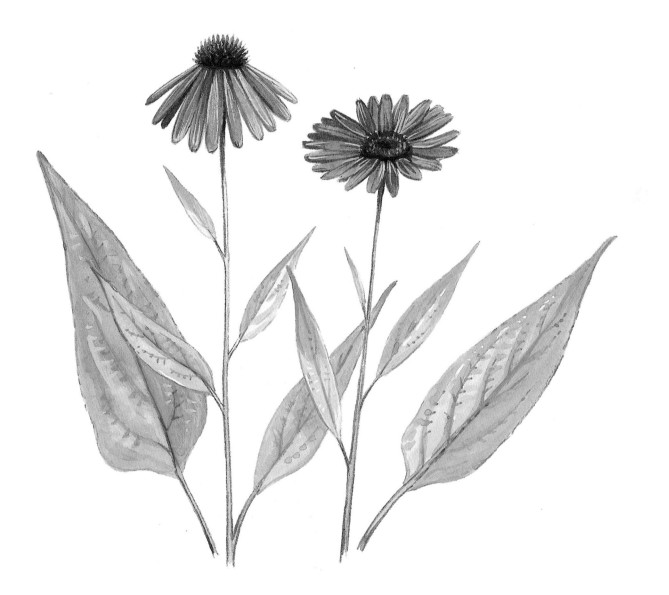

Echinacea, coneflower

Family Compositae/Asteraceae

ORIGIN AND CULTIVATION

There are nine indigenous North American *Echinacea* species, of which *E. purpurea, E. angustifolia,* and *E. pallida* are utilized for the preparation of herbal medicine; this is normally obtained from the roots and rhizomes, but sometimes also from the fresh flowering and dried aerial parts.

The plants grow wild in the prairies of North America, but there is also cultivation in Europe, North America, and Australia; the roots and rhizomes are lifted in the autumn. There is utilization of *Echinacea* species as ornamental plants. The flower heads have a pungent and acrid taste when chewed.

PLANT DESCRIPTION

Echinacea species are herbaceous perennials. *E. purpurea* may grow to a height of just over 1 m (3 ft), and has ovate, coarsely toothed leaves. Its flower heads (inflorescences) are purple (ray florets), with conical orange–brown centres (disc florets). *E. pallida* is of similar height but with narrow (lanceolate) leaves, and *E. angustifolia* is shorter.

CULINARY USES AND NUTRITIONAL VALUE

None.

CLAIMS AND FOLKLORE

From time immemorial the native North Americans used echinacea for the treatment of snakebite and wounds, and to relieve fever. It was adopted by the settlers, and in the late nineteenth and early twentieth centuries there were claims that the drug could relieve or cure many ailments.

The drug is now available in decoctions, infusions, liquid extracts, tablets, and other forms, on a world-wide basis. It is increasingly seen in cosmetics (e.g. lip balms, shampoos, toothpaste), and in health foods and herb teas; almost 300 different products are available in Europe.

Echinacea has two major uses. Applied externally, it is claimed to be effective in dealing with hard-to-heal wounds, eczema, burns, psoriasis, herpes, insect stings, and bites. Probably of more interest is its utilization as a non-specific stimulant of the immune system and, therefore, its possible use both as a prophylactic and a treatment in common infectious diseases, such as colds and influenza.

EVIDENCE

The root contains a variety of chemical substances, including high molecular weight polysaccharides, amides, glycosides, alkaloids, and essential oils. Some of the substances, can be used to distinguish between the three species normally utilized. The leaves contain similar substances, but in less quantity than the roots.

There have been a considerable number of animal and human studies into the efficacy of echinacea extracts. Some support has been provided for its use as a non-specific stimulant of the immune system, although more research would be advisable. A number of the chemical compounds present have been identified as immunostimulants, although not, as once thought, the glycoside echinacoside. There is also some experimental evidence supporting the use of echinacea ointment or extract in the treatment of insect bites or stings, and burns.

Echinacea shows little toxicity but, nevertheless, is not recommended for use during pregnancy.

In Germany, the use of *E. pallida* root and *E. purpurea* aerial parts and flower is supported, but not the aerial parts, flower, and root of *E. angustifolia*, or the aerial parts and flower of *E. pallida*. Sometimes, commercial preparations of *E. pallida* are incorrectly labelled '*Echinacea angustifolia*'.

Elder (European) *Sambucus nigra;*
elder (American) *S. canadensis*

Family Caprifoliaceae

ORIGIN AND CULTIVATION

Sambucus nigra is widely found in Europe, western Asia, and North Africa, growing in woods, waste places, and near buildings, and is often cultivated. It is naturalized in North America, where the native species is *S. canadensis*.

PLANT DESCRIPTION

European elder is a shrub or small tree growing to a height of about 10 m (33 ft); American elder grows to a height of about 4 m (13 ft). The branches of the plant have a brownish grey corky bark, and there is a large proportion of soft, light, whitish pith. Its leaves have 5–7 – toothed leaflets. The creamy white flowers give rise to purplish black fruit.

Herbal products are normally obtained from the flowers.

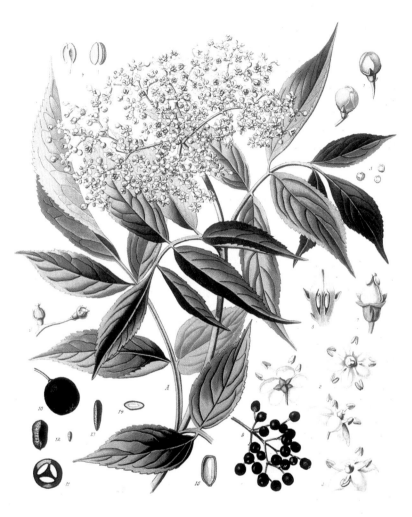

CULINARY AND NUTRITIONAL VALUE

Elder flowers (actually the petals) are used to make still or sparkling (not to be described as 'champagne') wine and cordial, a preserve with gooseberries, and, with the addition of flour and egg, fritters. The berries are used to make wine, and added to apple pies or apple and blackberry jellies. It is considered safe to use the berries, particularly when cooked, but the roots, stems, and leaves are said to contain a poisonous alkaloid and glycoside, which cause nausea, vomiting, and diarrhoea, so these plant parts should not be included in food products.

CLAIMS AND FOLKLORE

Elder extracts have traditionally been used to treat influenza, colds, and catarrh, and are said to have diaphoretic, diuretic, and laxative properties. Extracts are also included in skin lotions, oils, and ointments.

EVIDENCE

Analysis has shown a wide range of chemical compounds in elder. It has been stated that flavonoids and triterpenes are the active principles. There have been a considerable number of animal experiments, but no documented human studies. The animal experiments seem to support the reported anti-inflammatory, antiviral, and diuretic properties of elder.

Elder should not be used during pregnancy and lactation. It is supported in Germany.

Evening primrose *Oenothera biennis*

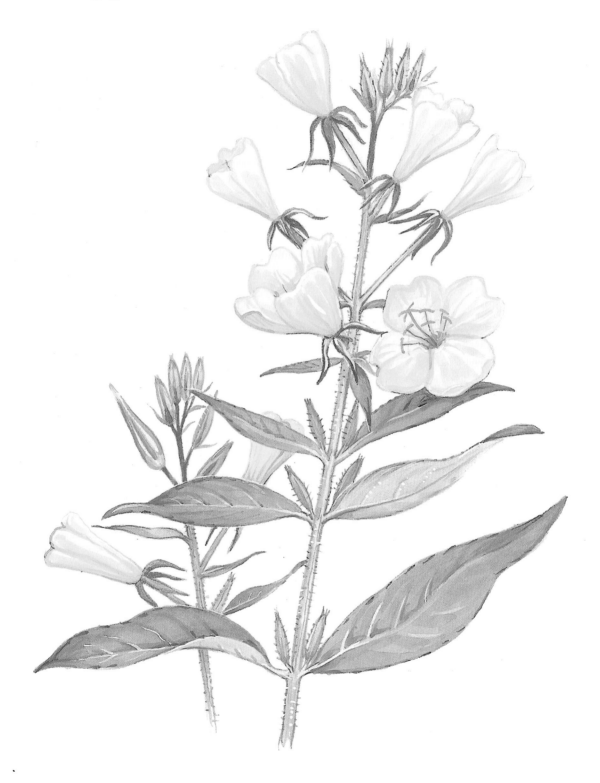

Evening primrose

Family Onagraceae

ORIGIN AND CULTIVATION

Oenothera biennis is native to North America, but is cultivated there and in at least 15 European countries. The plant is grown for its seed, the source of an important oil. It is cultivated either as an annual or a biennial. Evening primrose has been subjected to intensive plant breeding to produce more effective cultivars.

PLANT DESCRIPTION

It grows to a height of 30–150 cm (5 ft), with a basal rosette of lance-shaped leaves 10–22 cm (9 in) long and 1 cm ($\frac{2}{5}$ in) wide. The yellow flowers give rise to dry pods containing numerous minute seeds.

CULINARY AND NUTRITIONAL VALUE

The leaves, shoots, root, and seeds have been used as food by the North American Indians.

CLAIMS AND FOLKLORE

Evening primrose oil has long been available as a dietary supplement. It has been used to treat atopic eczema, mastalgia, premenstrual and menopausal syndromes, acne, brittle nails, hyperactivity in children, rheumatoid arthritis, coronary artery disease, alcohol-related liver damage, and multiple sclerosis.

Externally, it has been claimed to be effective for dry skin, and has been included in hand lotions, soaps, shampoos, and other cosmetic products.

Infusions of the leaves and stem have been used to treat asthma, gastrointestinal disorders, whooping cough, and certain female complaints.

EVIDENCE

The seed contains about 14% fatty oil, which is made up of 50–70% linoleic acid, 7–10% gamma-linolenic acid, and small quantities of other acids. Linoleic acid and gamma-linolenic acid are 'essential' fatty acids, necessary as cellular structural elements, and as precursors of prostaglandins, chemicals important in the body metabolism. Essential fatty acids cannot be made in the body but must be taken in the diet. Evening primrose oil can therefore be an important source of essential fatty acids, in particular gamma-linolenic acid. Generally speaking, the oil is most useful for dealing with atopic eczema. Some evidence supports its use in treating premenstrual syndrome, mastalgia, diabetic neuropathy, rheumatoid arthritis, renal disease, irritable bowel syndrome, and ulcerative colitis, and in reducing blood cholesterol and blood pressure in coronary heart disease. Clearly, the therapeutic value of the oil is worthy of further research.

The oil is virtually non-toxic, although it might be wise to avoid it during pregnancy.

Eyebright *Euphrasia officinalis*

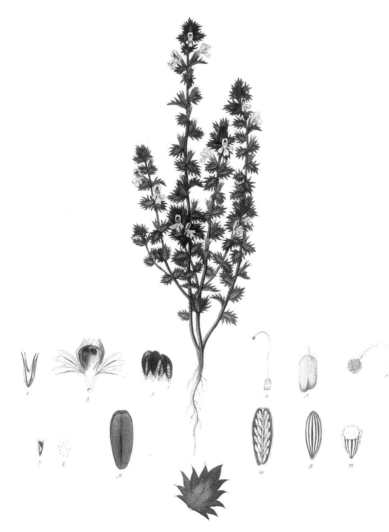

Family Scrophulariaceae

ORIGIN AND CULTIVATION

Euphrasia contains a large number of species that are semiparasitic and therefore difficult to cultivate. They are found in the cold temperate regions of the Northern and Southern Hemispheres, occupying a variety of habitats. *E. officinalis* is found in pastures and grasslands, being parasitic on plants such as clover, plantain, and grasses.

PLANT DESCRIPTION

Eyebright is an annual that varies tremendously in height, according to its habitat, from 3 to 30 cm (1 ft). Its leaves are small, ovate, and deeply toothed. The small white or reddish flowers are streaked with purple, and there is a yellow spot in the throat.

CULINARY AND NUTRITIONAL VALUE

None.

CLAIMS AND FOLKLORE

Eyebright has probably been used in herbal medicine since the time of Theophrastus, in the third or fourth century BC. It has been utilized for a number of conditions, such as allergies, cancers, coughs, skin diseases, and others. However, most attention has been concentrated on its value as a treatment for eye conditions (hence the name of the plant) such as conjunctivitis. According to the medieval Doctrine of Signatures, the flower resembled a diseased eye and therefore the plant would be suitable for the treatment of such diseases. This belief is still held by some today.

EVIDENCE

Eyebright contains a variety of chemical substances, including iridoid and other glycosides, and tannins. There seems to be little scientific evidence to support the herbal use of the plant. Indeed, its use for the treatment for eye diseases is strongly discouraged in Germany.

It should be avoided during pregnancy and lactation.

Fennel *Foeniculum vulgare*

Family Umbelliferae/Apiaceae

ORIGIN AND CULTIVATION

Fennel is a native of the Mediterranean area but has become naturalized throughout much of Europe. It is cultivated in a number of countries, including India, and was originally introduced to North America by the Spanish and British.

PLANT DESCRIPTION

The plant is a perennial herb, up to 2 m (6 ft) in height, with thread-like leaf segments 1–5 cm (2 in) in length. Its yellow flowers are held in umbels and give rise to 'seeds' (botanically speaking, fruits), about 4 mm ($\frac{1}{6}$ in) long, which are oblong–ovoid, flattened, greenish or yellowish brown, or greyish, with yellow ridges.

The parts used are the 'seeds' or essential oil.

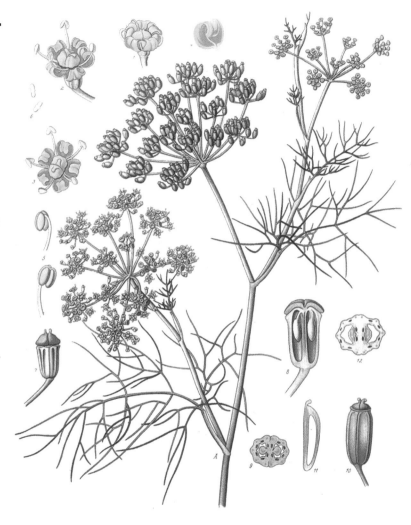

CULINARY AND NUTRITIONAL VALUE

The 'seeds' produce 3–6% of an aromatic essential oil, the main constituent of which is anethole. Either the 'seed' or the oil are used to flavour bread, pastries, confectionery, liqueurs, and fish dishes. The leaves are employed as a garnish and flavour for fish. Florence or Florentine fennel (*Foeniculum vulgare* var. *dulce*) has swollen leaf bases that can be cooked or eaten raw in salads. These leaf bases contain 95% water; little protein, fat, or sugar; a large amount of potassium and a range of minerals; carotenes, vitamins E and the B complex, and a small amount of vitamin C.

CLAIMS AND FOLKLORE

Extracts of fennel 'seeds' have been used as a carminative and stomachic, and have been utilized to increase lactation, pro-mote menstruation, and increase libido. They have also been included in cough preparations, and in colic-relieving medicines for infants.

EVIDENCE

The essential oil produced by the 'seed' has already been mentioned. Animal experiments and human studies have shown this to be antispasmodic. Possibly this explains the reported carminative properties of fennel.

Fennel 'seed' preparations seem to have no toxic effects if used in normal herbal medicines, except possibly for the odd allergic reaction, but ingestion of the essential oil can have quite serious effects and therefore should be avoided.

It is supported in Germany.

Feverfew *Tanacetum parthenium syn. Chrysanthemum parthenium*

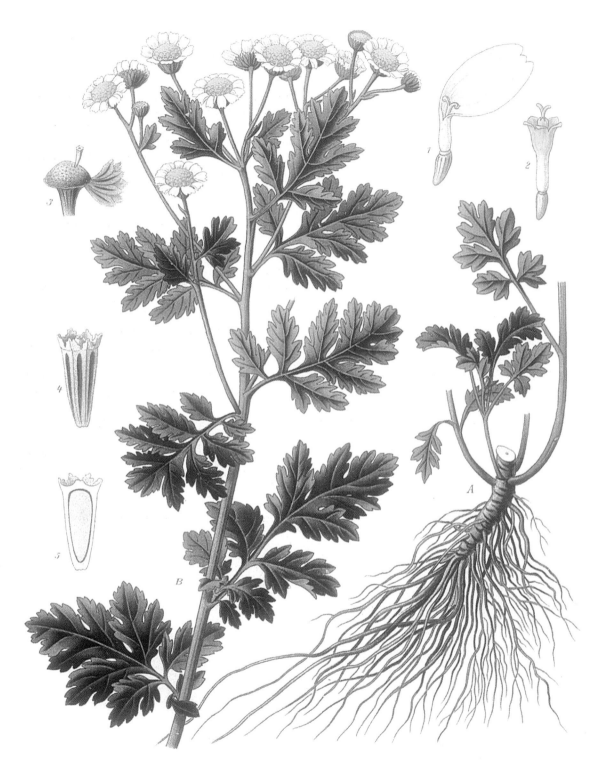

Feverfew

Family Compositae/Asteraceae

ORIGIN AND CULTIVATION

Feverfew probably originated in southern and eastern Europe, but is now common throughout Europe, Australia, and North America. It grows well in scrubland, rocky and waste places, and hedges, and is often a sign of poor soil quality. Feverfew has long been cultivated as an ornamental or medicinal plant.

PLANT DESCRIPTION

It is a perennial growing to a height of 45 cm (18 in) or more, with strong smelling, greenish yellow, feather-like leaves. The daisy-like inflorescences are 1 cm ($\frac{1}{2}$ in) across, and are arranged spirally around the main stem, with the stalks of the lower inflorescences elongated so that the top of the entire flower head is nearly flat (a corymb). Each inflorescence is made up of central yellow disc florets and a single layer of outer white ray florets. A number of horticultural cultivars and varieties exist.

CULINARY USES AND NUTRITIONAL VALUE

Feverfew has been used as a herb in cooking, but only in moderation because of its bitter taste.

CLAIMS AND FOLKLORE

The plant has a long history in traditional and folk medicine. Since Roman times it has been used to induce menstruation, and to aid placenta expulsion in child birth. As the common name suggests, feverfew has been utilized to lower body temperature (an antipyretic), and it has been put to a vast number of other uses.

More modern work has suggested that feverfew might act as an antispasmodic, antibiotic, and antithrombotic agent, and be toxic to human tumour cells. However, most attention has been given to the value of the leaf (and possibly the stem) in treating and preventing migraine and, to a lesser extent, arthritis and rheumatism.

It has also been suggested that feverfew might be planted around houses to 'purify' the air with its strong odour, and a tincture of the flowers doubles as an insect repellent and a balm for bites.

EVIDENCE

The active chemical constituents in the leaf (and stem) are sesquiterpene lactones, and parthenolide, particularly, appears to inhibit release of the hormone serotonin, which is thought to trigger migraine, although there is no universal agreement. There is considerable clinical and experimental evidence to support its use as an anti-migraine agent, although it should not be taken for more than 4 months without medical advice. It is officially approved in Canada and may be taken as fresh or dried leaves, capsules, or tablets.

There is not much experimental evidence to support its use against rheumatism or arthritis.

Side-effects may include mouth ulcers and gastrointestinal disturbance, and it should not be taken by pregnant or lactating mothers, or children under 2 years. Those who are allergic to members of the Compositae/Asteraceae family (e.g. daisy, chrysanthemum) should take care.

Fish oils

There are two different types of fish oils – those that come from the liver of 'lean' fish such as cod, and those that are extracted from the flesh of fatty fish such as mackerel, herring, or salmon. Fish oils have a high content of fatty acids, with 20 or more carbon chains that are either predominantly monounsaturated, or polyunsaturated with five or six double bonds belonging to the n-3 family (see p. xvi). Fish liver oils also contain large amounts of vitamins A and D and are available as oil or in capsules as a dietary supplement of these vitamins. Fish body oils are usually purified and supplements do not generally contain the vitamins.

Many years ago it was observed that Greenland Inuit had a low incidence of coronary heart disease despite their high fat and cholesterol intakes. Most of the fat was from marine foods, with large quantities of the long-chain n-3 fatty acids eicosapentanoate (EPA) and docosahexanoate (DHA) and research has now demonstrated that these fatty acids affect blood clotting mechanisms so that blood clots that might block coronary arteries narrowed by atherosclerosis are less likely to form. These effects are seen with purified fish oils as well as when fatty fish are consumed. In the UK it had previously been recommended that adults consume two to three portions of fatty fish each week, but fish consumption is generally much lower than this. Recently the UK Food Standards Agency recommended that only two portions of fish, one white and one oily, be eaten per week. Shark, swordfish, and marlin may be contaminated with mercury and should not be eaten by pregnant women, women who intend to become pregnant, and infants and children under 16. Purified fish oils represent a way of obtaining the n-3 fatty acids, but care should be taken to keep to recommended doses. As with plant foods, the foods themselves may contain other, as yet unknown, substances that could also have important effects.

The Joint Health Claims Initiative has assessed the evidence that consumption of the types of long-chain fatty acids found in fish oils benefits heart health and in 2005 agreed that foods containing these may use the following generic claim. *'Eating 3g weekly, or 0.45g daily, long chain omega-3 polyunsaturated fatty acids, as part of a healthy lifestyle, helps maintain heart health.'*

Important caveats to the use of the claim are that it relates only to very long chain polyunsaturated fatty acids (of chain length 20 carbons or above) including EPA, and DHA, and not all long chain polyunsaturated fatty acids, such as alpha-linolenic acid (which have chain lengths of less than 20). The ratio of EPA and DHA should reflect that which occurs naturally in oily fish' and include the statement that *'The Government advises that at least 2 servings of fish, one of which should be oily, containing approximately 3g LC n-3 PUFA, is consumed each week'* Manufacturers of supplements should also point out that oily fish is an alternative supplier of the long-chain n-3 fatty acids. The Food and Drug Administration in the USA has also allowed a qualified health claim for n-3 fatty acids and heart health.

There has been much recent interest in the idea that supplements of long-chain n-3 fatty acids may improve behaviour and reading and spelling ability in some children, specifically those with a condition called developmental coordination disorder. Although there is evidence that these fatty acids are important in pre-natal brain development and for post-natal development in premature infants more research is needed to clarify the possible cognitive benefits in older children and in the elderly.

Some studies have suggested that consumption of long-chain n-3 polyunsaturated fatty acids may help protect against diabetes (incidence is lower in populations with high fatty fish intakes), and may lower blood pressure in patients with hypertension. Fish oil supplements (fish liver oils as well as fish body oils) have been shown in some studies to reduce pain and inflammation in rheumatoid arthritis, although more research is needed here. Trials of fish oils in the treatment of skin diseases such as atopic (allergic) eczema and psoriasis have shown mixed results. Fish oils do not seem to have much effect on eczema, but they have been shown to have modest beneficial effects on psoriasis, especially when taken in conjunction with other treatments, as they may alleviate some of the side-effects of drug treatments. *If you are receiving medical treatment for any of these disorders it is advisable to see your doctor before consuming fish oil supplements.*

Garlic *Allium sativum*

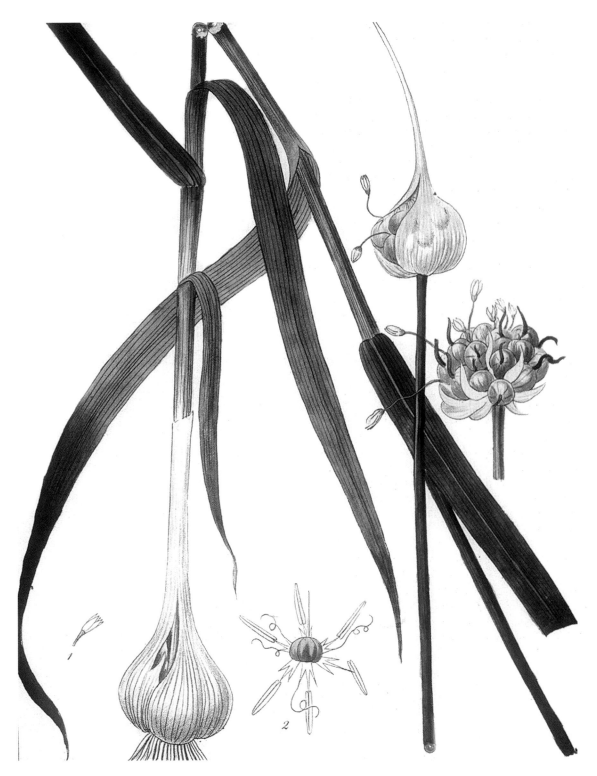

Garlic

Family Liliaceae

ORIGIN AND CULTIVATION

Garlic is not known in the wild and probably evolved from the wild *Allium longicuspis* of central Asia. The plant spread to the Mediterranean region in ancient times, being known in Egypt from at least 3000 BC. It is also an ancient crop in India and China. Spanish, Portuguese, and French settlers introduced the plant to the New World.

The crop grows easily in cool and warm climates, and is now found all over the world; the leading producers are China, South Korea, India, Spain, and the USA.

PLANT DESCRIPTION

The main part utilized is the underground bulb, which is up to 7 cm (3 in) in diameter, but the aerial leaves and flowering stem are also sometimes included in food, particularly in South-east Asia.

The bulb consists of a number of segments, or 'cloves' (4–15 cm), enclosed in white, pinkish, or even purple dry outer scales of the original parent bulb.

At maturity, the plant is 30–60 cm (2 ft) tall, with linear and flat leaves, 1–2.5 cm (1 in) broad. Inflorescences, which are not always produced, consist of umbels of white or pinkish flowers (3–4 mm in length), usually mixed up with small aerial bulbs and enclosed in whitish, long, and pointed coverings or spathes. The plant does not set fertile seed. Propagation is entirely by vegetative means. Single cloves are set firmly in the ground in sandy soil – in the spring in climates with a cold winter and in autumn in Mediterranean climates. The first bulbs harvested may be single and solid, but if replanted the following spring they produce large and multicloved bulbs.

CULINARY AND NUTRITIONAL VALUE

Garlic is one of the world's best known flavouring agents. It is rarely used as a vegetable but is included in some dishes, e.g. 'Provençal 40 clove chicken'. Garlic as a flavouring agent is used in many dishes and products (e.g. salads, sauces, spaghetti, soups, curries, garlic bread, garlic butter, meats, sausages); it can also act as a preservative in the forms of mince, juice, dehydrated powder, or distilled oil.

The bulb contains about 8% protein, 15% starch, small amounts of fat and sugars, a range of minerals, with large amounts of potassium (620 mg per 100 g) and phosphorus (170 mg per 100 g), a range of B vitamins, vitamin E, and vitamin C (17 mg per 100 g); the energy content is 98 kcal (411 kJ) per 100 g.

CLAIMS AND FOLKLORE

Since ancient times, various cures have been attributed to garlic. It has been used as an antidote to snake and scorpion bites; as a cold cure, by rubbing the soles of the feet with 'cloves'; to cure athlete's foot, by placing 'cloves' between the toes; to ward off witches and vampires; to prevent ageing; and to treat the plague.

As a herbal medicine, garlic has been and is used to treat chronic bronchitis, respiratory catarrh, recurrent colds, whooping cough, bronchitic asthma, influenza, and other health problems. It is marketed in the form of capsules, extracts, and tablets.

EVIDENCE

The bulb contains alliin (allylcysteine sulphoxide), which is odourless. When the bulb tissue is disrupted, enzyme action converts alliin into an odoriferous essential oil (0.1–0.36% of the bulb) containing a number of sulphur compounds such as allicin (diallyl thiosulphinate), allyl-propyl disulphide, and others.

A considerable number of scientific investigations, together with epidemiological evidence, concerning humans and animals have supported the medical value of garlic and its products: (a) it is effective against some bacteria (e.g. *Staphylococcus, Salmonella*) and some fungi (e.g. *Trichophyton, Candida albicans*), and may have antiviral activity; (b) there is some evidence from animal studies that garlic can suppress cancer initiation and development; (c) it reduces blood sugar, triglycerides (fats), and high blood pressure; (d) it reduces blood cholesterol and improves the high-density lipoprotein to low-density lipoprotein ratio; (e) it has an antithrombotic (blood clotting) effect and an antiplatelet aggregation effect; and (f) it can act as a vermifuge.

It is generally agreed that garlic is non-toxic, and clearly a strong body of scientific evidence supports its health value in relation to cardiovascular problems and infections; however, therapeutic doses of garlic may interfere with existing anticoagulant therapies.

The odour of garlic is offensive to some people. Consequently, so-called 'odourless' products have been developed, but not much seems to be known about the effect of the deodorization process on the active principles.

Fresh garlic is supported in Germany.

Ginger *Zingiber officinale*

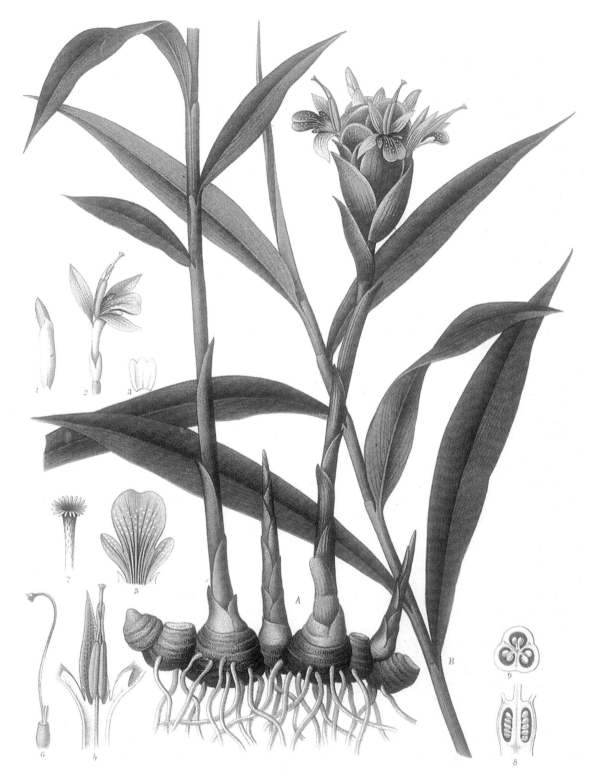

Ginger

Family Zingiberaceae

ORIGIN AND CULTIVATION

Ginger evolved in South-east Asia but is never found in the wild state. It has been used as a spice and medicine in India and China since ancient times; it was known to the Greeks and Romans and generally throughout Europe by the tenth century. Today it can be found in cultivation in most tropical countries; Jamaica, India, Nigeria, Sierra Leone, Australia, and China are well known sources.

PLANT DESCRIPTION

Ginger is a perennial herb 30–100 cm (3 ft) in height, with an underground stem (rhizome) with swollen segments. The aerial stem has narrow, sword-shaped leaves. Flowers are rarely seen but, if present, are yellowish or greenish white.

The rhizome, often erroneously referred to as the root, is the part used.

CULINARY AND NUTRITIONAL VALUE

The plant is of great importance as a spice or flavouring agent, being included in biscuits, puddings, cakes, ginger-bread, soups, pickles, curry powder, ginger beer, ginger ale, and ginger wine. For these purposes, the rhizome itself may be utilized, or its essential oil or its oleoresin, a solvent extraction of the rhizome, which contains other substances in addition to the oil.

CLAIMS AND FOLKLORE

Ginger has had many uses in herbal medicine. It is said to be carminative, and has been used for hundreds of years to treat gastrointestinal distress. It is also employed as an antipyretic, diuretic, diaphoretic, and antitussive (stops coughing) – these properties would explain its use for colds and influenza. It is claimed that ginger stimulates the circulation and helps blood flow to the surface, useful for chilblains and poor circulation to the hands and feet.

EVIDENCE

There have been a considerable number of animal and human experiments into the therapeutic value of ginger. Many of its traditional uses have been supported. Essential oil and gingerols and their derivatives (shogaols) present in the oleoresin are regarded as the active principles.

Some animal experiments indicate that ginger shows cardiotonic activity (favourable action on the heart). The essential oil has been demonstrated as antibacterial, at least *in vitro*.

There has been considerable interest in ginger as an agent for calming travel or motion sickness. Some human studies support this use, but not all.

In Germany, it has been recommended as a treatment for dyspepsia and motion sickness.

Excessive doses should be avoided during pregnancy and lactation, and by those suffering from, eg., cardiac or diabetic conditions.

Ginkgo, maidenhair tree *Ginkgo biloba*

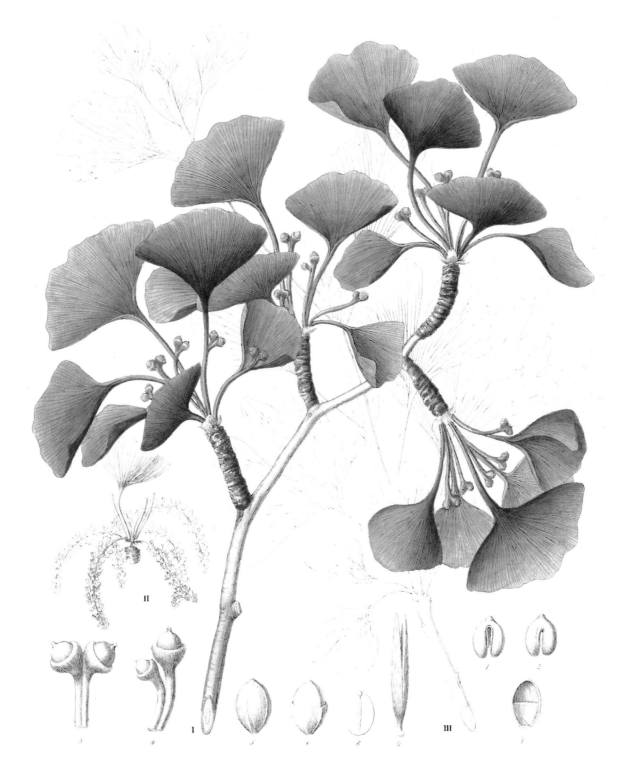

Ginkgo, maidenhair tree

Family Ginkgoaceae

ORIGIN AND CULTIVATION

Ginkgo is a member of the gymnosperms, plants with seeds that are exposed, rather than enclosed in fruits as in the angiosperms. The species is the sole survivor of a group of trees, which, in early geological times, was almost cosmopolitan. Direct ancestors of the tree existed in many parts of the world before the beginning of the Jurassic period (about 180 million years ago). It has sometimes been described as a 'living fossil'.

Probably the species no longer exists in the truly wild state. It is a sacred tree in the Far East, being commonly planted in the grounds of temples and palaces; some specimens are reputed to be over 1000 years old. Because of the present day interest in ginkgo as a herbal product and for urban planting, it is now cultivated in large-scale plantations in China, France, and North Carolina and Maryland in the USA, and no doubt other places. The trees are good for urban planting because they can withstand high levels of pollution and low levels of sunlight.

PLANT DESCRIPTION

Ginkgo is a deciduous tree up to 35 m (120 ft) in height and 1 m (3 ft) in trunk diameter. The stalked leaves have fan-shaped blades 5–7 cm (3 in) across, with an apical notch. They superficially resemble the leaves of the maidenhair fern. The male and female flowers are borne on separate trees, and the seed (often erroneously referred to as a 'fruit') is about 3 cm (1 in) across and with a fleshy covering. A disadvantage with ginkgo as an urban tree is that the female produces seed, which gives off an unpleasant smell when it drops.

CULINARY AND NUTRITIONAL VALUE

The kernels of the seed are edible, with about 10% protein, 2.5% fat, and 67% starch. In China and Japan they are often eaten roasted at weddings and feasts, and are supposed to aid digestion and diminish the effects of drinking too much wine. On the other hand, contact or ingestion of the fleshy covering of the seed may lead to severe allergic reactions, including blisters. It is reported that the seed contains a toxic substance that is responsible for 'gin-nan' food poisoning in China and Japan. However, as stated earlier, the roasted kernel is quite a popular food item in the Orient; toxicity of the seed is related to excess taken during food shortages.

CLAIMS AND FOLKLORE

Ginkgo (both leaves and seeds) has been recorded in Chinese herbals from almost 5000 years ago, and has traditionally been used in the treatment of asthma, coughs, vaginal discharge, a weak bladder, and incontinence, and 'to benefit the brain'.

In relatively recent times, the leaf extract has become a best-selling herbal product in Western countries, with claims that it helps blood circulation (especially to the brain) and asthma. Improvement of blood circulation to the brain might alleviate the problem of diminishing mental and physical health with the onset of old age, by slowing down brain deterioration and offering some protection against strokes, memory loss, and tinnitus.

EVIDENCE

The key chemical constituents are flavonoids (flavonol glycosides and biflavones), diterpenes (ginkgolides), and sesquiterpenes (bilobalides).

Over the past 30 years a large number of clinical and scientific trials on humans and animals have been carried out, and they are continuing. In many cases, ginkgo extracts standardized to 24% flavonoid glycosides and 6% terpenoids have been utilized – other substances, e.g. ginkgolic acids, have been reduced to minute amounts. These acids are potent contact allergens, and this illustrates the necessity of standardizing herbal extracts. In Germany three different ginkgo extracts are reported, but only one is supported.

Some experiments support the claim that leaf extracts increase the blood flow to the brain (and the limbs) and scavenge free radicals that could affect brain cells. A great deal of attention has been paid to the action of the leaf extract, which has been demonstrated to be a potent antagonist to the platelet activating factor. This action could also inhibit brain cell deterioration and, in addition, be useful in the treatment of asthma and inflammation.

There is much confidence as regards the value of ginkgo in the treatment of some aspects of geriatric illness; indeed, an enormous number of prescriptions for the drug are given by physicians in Germany.

Korean (or Chinese) ginseng *Panax ginseng;*
Siberian ginseng *Eleutherococcus senticosus;*
American ginseng *Panax quinquefolius*

Family Araliaceae

ORIGIN AND CULTIVATION
Ginseng refers to a number of species and, in all cases, the herbal product is derived from the dried root.

- Korean or Chinese ginseng (*Panax ginseng*) has been used in Chinese medicine for at least 5000 years and is widely cultivated in Korea and China. There are two main commercial forms: (a) 'red' – the root is steamed after collection and before drying; and (b) 'white' – the root is dried immediately after collection and frequently the outer layer is removed.

  Some other *Panax* species are utilized in the East. One species, described as *P. pseudoginseng,* was utilized by the Vietcong during the Vietnam war to assist the healing of those suffering from gunshot wounds.

  P. ginseng was introduced into Europe several times from the ninth century onwards, but assumed no importance in Western medicine until relatively recent times.

- Siberian ginseng (*Eleutherococcus senticosus*) was developed by Russian scientists in the 1950s as an alternative to *P. ginseng.*

- American ginseng (*P. quinquefolius*) is a native of northeastern America. It was once abundant in the wild but is now a threatened, rare, or endangered species, and therefore the harvesting of the root is subject to monitoring. Cultivation takes place in the USA, Canada, and China. The plant was 'discovered' by Jesuits in the eighteenth century, and first collected by backwoodsmen for export to China, where it was described in traditional medicine in about 1765.

PLANT DESCRIPTION
- Korean or Chinese ginseng: an herbaceous perennial with a carrot-like root and an upright stem with a whorl of 2–5 divided leaves. The small green–yellow flowers are arranged in umbels (the flower stalks are positioned like the ribs of an umbrella) and give rise to red berries. The height of the plant is up to 90 cm (3 ft).

- Siberian ginseng: a deciduous shrub up to 3 m (10 ft) in height, with dark green, divided leaves and numerous thin thorns. The flowers are unisexual, in umbels, with lilac–purple males and green females giving rise to blue–black berries.

- American ginseng: rather similar to *P. ginseng.*

CLAIMS AND FOLKLORE
The types of ginseng have been used primarily as prophylactic drugs rather than remedial preparations. Ginseng is described as an 'adaptogen', which is a drug that increases non-specific resistance (i.e. an immunostimulant action) of an organism to infection and stress, helps prevent fatigue, and acts as a tonic in convalescence or cases of general exhaustion.

Ginseng is available as the crude herb, powdered root, tea, liquid extracts, capsules, and tablets.

It is also available in cosmetic products (lotions, creams, soaps, etc.), but the scientific reason for this is not immediately obvious.

EVIDENCE
The active principles in *Panax* ginsengs are thought to be triterpenoid saponins known as 'ginsenosides'. In contrast, Siberian ginseng contains hardly any saponins, and the activity is ascribed to 'eleutherosides'. In both *Panax* and Siberian ginseng, it would appear that these active principles work best in conjunction with each other in a mixture. The polysaccharides present in the root might contribute to the immunostimulant action of ginseng.

Many experiments with both animals and humans have investigated the effects of ginseng. There seems to be some support for its adaptogenic (immunostimulant) properties. Some other uses have also been suggested, e.g. treatment of cancer and diabetes, although these are less well accepted. In support of these experiments, one must also bear in mind the appreciation of the value of ginseng that has extended over thousands of years.

However, a number of areas require further investigation. The suggested dosages vary according to the authority. Also, based on traditional medicine: (a) the drug should not be taken by children, healthy adults under 40 years of age, pregnant women, and those suffering from diabetes or hypertension; (b) the middle-aged should take ginseng on intermittent courses, i.e., there should be root-free periods; (c) the use of other stimulants, e.g. amphetamines and caffeine, should be avoided;

Korean (or Chinese) ginseng, Siberian ginseng, American ginseng

(d) ginseng should not be given to those undergoing hypoglycaemic, hypotensive, and steroid therapy; and (e) the elderly and chronically sick can take low (0.4–0.8 g) doses on a regular basis. However, according to another system, ginseng may be taken by the 'young and healthy'. There is also the problem that commercial preparations are not necessarily standardized according to the active principles.

Generally speaking, ginseng has low acute toxicity, but long-term use may lead to hypertension and insomnia. It is supported in Germany.

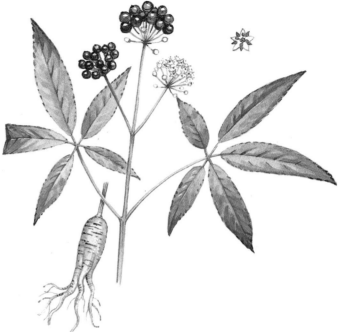

Korean or Chinese ginseng.

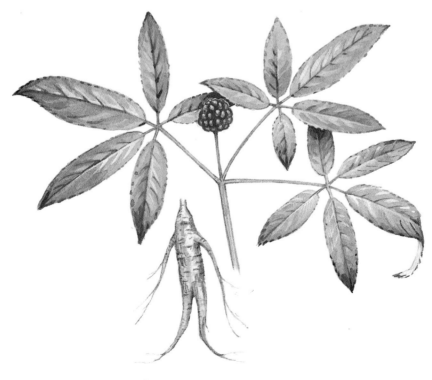

American ginseng.

Glucosamine (sulphate) and chondroitin (sulphate)

ORIGIN

These are fairly new supplements, and are extracted from crab shells and cow cartilage (windpipes).

CULINARY AND NUTRITIONAL VALUE

None.

CLAIMS AND FOLKLORE

Cartilage assists in the easy movement of joints, and its degeneration leads to osteoarthritis, the most common form of arthritis and a leading cause of disability. Non-steroidal, anti-inflammatory drugs are used to alleviate the pain of this illness, although there is a fear that they might have toxic effects, particularly in the elderly population.

Because both glucosamine and chondroitin contribute to the structure of cartilage (articular), they have been given as supplements to treat the pain of osteoarthritis, and hopefully slow down the progress of the disease. They have also been investigated as possible substitutes for non-steroidal anti-inflammatory drugs.

EVIDENCE

The results of animal and human (double blind with a placebo) studies are encouraging. Osteoarthritis in the knee joint has been investigated, and one recent clinical study using glucosamine sulphate as a painkiller found it effective with patients suffering from mild to moderate pain. Investigations suggest that these supplements have few side-effects, although it has been suggested that diabetic and overweight persons should exercise caution with the supplements. The results are encouraging, but it is generally understood that there is a need for long-term studies into efficacy, purity of the supplements, and dosages, although these considerations apply to all supplements.

It is possible that glucosamine (and chondroitin) might slow the rate of cartilage deterioration, but it is not likely that they will replace lost cartilage.

These supplements are used extensively in many countries and patients are very supportive as regards the treatment.

Goldenseal *Hydrastis canadensis*

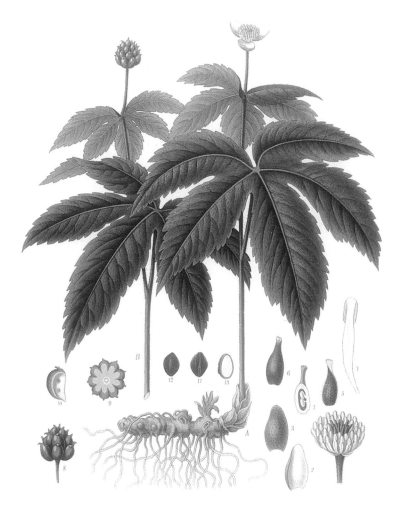

Family Ranunculaceae

ORIGIN AND CULTIVATION

Goldenseal grows wild in certain parts of North America, but overharvesting has led to scarcity. Because of this, there is now some official control. Cultivation is practised but the product is expensive.

PLANT DESCRIPTION

The plant is an herbaceous perennial growing to a height of about 30 cm (1 ft). There is a horizontal rhizome that is brown externally and yellow inside. The leaves are five-lobed, and a plant produces a single insignificant flower that develops into a red fruit.

The rhizome is the source of the herbal drug.

CULINARY AND NUTRITIONAL VALUE

None.

CLAIMS AND FOLKLORE

Goldenseal was used by the native North Americans, and then by the settlers, almost as a 'cure-all' – to treat wounds, ulcers, inflamed eyes, and, internally, stomach and liver problems. Modern herbalists consider extracts astringent and antibacterial, suitable for dealing with the mucous membranes of the body. Consequently, it has been used as an eyewash, a mouthwash for infected gums, and as a douche for vaginal infections. Similarly, it has been suggested as a treatment for inflamed mucous membranes lining the gut. In addition, it is said to reduce heavy menstrual bleeding, and to help stop bleeding following childbirth.

EVIDENCE

The active principles in goldenseal are said to be alkaloids (isoquinoline), of which two are berberine and hydrastine. A few animal experiments have been carried out to test the efficacy of goldenseal, but no human studies, although berberine and hydrastine have been well investigated.

It is difficult to come to a final judgement concerning the therapeutic value of goldenseal. Some people do not support it at all; others feel that it can be used in a modest manner to relieve some skin problems, whereas modern herbalists describe a number of functions. However, all would agree that excessive use should be avoided, and that it should not be given to those with high blood pressure and not consumed during pregnancy and lactation.

Goldenseal extracts, it has been alleged, mask positive results when urine is tested for illicit drugs. There is no scientific evidence to support this claim.

Guarana *Paullinia cupana syn. P. sorbilis*

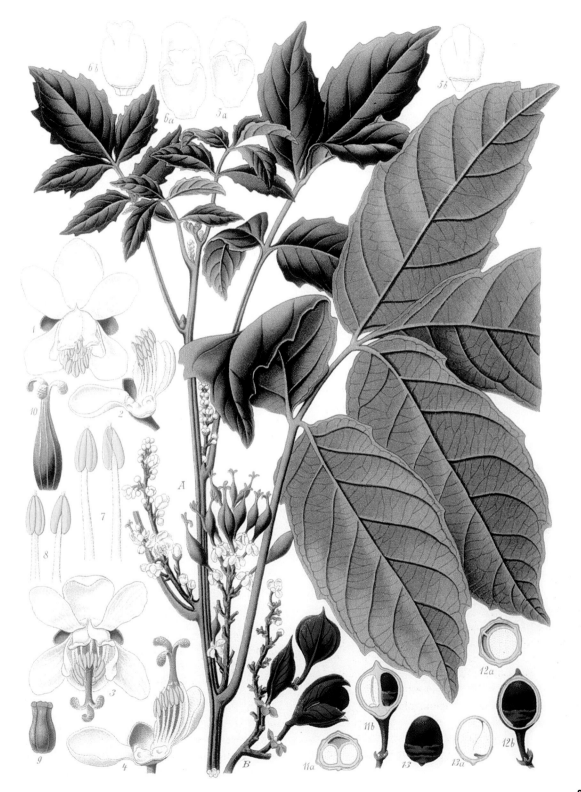

Guarana

Family Sapindaceae

ORIGIN AND CULTIVATION
Guarana is a climbing evergreen plant native to the Amazon region of South America (e.g. Brazil, Venezuela). It is commercially produced in the middle Amazon area of northern Brazil, with the city and county of Maués accounting for 80% of the world's supply.

PLANT DESCRIPTION
The plant has pinnately divided leaves with toothed margins and inconspicuous yellow flowers in spikes up to 10 cm (4 in) in length. These give rise to red capsules that open when ripe to expose 1–3 shining purple–brown seeds. In the natural situation, guarana grows to a height of about 10 m (33 ft) but under cultivation it forms a shrub about 2 m (7 ft) high.

CULINARY AND NUTRITIONAL VALUE
The seeds are pulverized, roasted, and then mixed with water to form a paste that is moulded into bars or cylinders and finally dried.

The active constituent is the alkaloid caffeine (3–5% of the dry weight), together with some related alkaloids. Other constituents include tannins (about 12%). The caffeine found in guarana was once referred to as 'guaranine', but is now known to be identical with the caffeine of coffee beans (1–2%) and tea leaves (1–4%). Because of its caffeine content, guarana acts as a stimulant, relieving physical and mental fatigue.

It is widely used to flavour cola, liqueurs, cordials, and confectionery, with levels usually below 0.002%. In Brazil a carbonated soft drink (offered commercially since 1909) is made from the seeds and considered a national beverage. Guarana is found in health foods, herb teas, tablets, capsules, chewing gum, slimming foods, and supplements for athletes (related to its value as a stimulant).

CLAIMS AND FOLKLORE
Guarana has been used by the natives of South America for a long time as a stimulant, an astringent, to protect against malaria, to treat chronic diarrhoea, and as an aphrodisiac. It was first noted by a Jesuit missionary in 1669, and by the eighteenth century its use had spread widely in Brazil. Commercial plantations were established in the 1970s and it is now a major cash crop. Guarana has played an important part in certain social aspects of South American natives, often being taken during periods of fast to increase tolerance to dietary restrictions.

Extracts of the stems, leaves, and roots have been used as a fish-killing drug in Central and South America. Stems of the closely related *Paullinia yoco* have been used by the native people of Colombia, Equador, and northern Peru to make a drink similar to guarana.

EVIDENCE
Guarana, because of its caffeine content, clearly acts as a stimulant. It has been claimed that it has a more sustained effect than tea or coffee, which may be related to the interaction of its caffeine with other substances present, e.g. tannins. Guarana is not recommended for people with cardiovascular disease, hypertension, or gastric ulcers. Mild expressions of caffeine overdose have been encountered because products containing guarana have not indicated the presence of caffeine. Excessive intake of guarana leads to symptoms such as excitability, restlessness, increased diuresis, headache, and possibly tremor or palpitations; these symptoms are associated with caffeine overdose.

The daily dose of powdered guarana should not exceed 3 g.

Hawthorn Crataegus oxyacanthoides, C. monogyna

Family Rosaceae

ORIGIN AND CULTIVATION

Hawthorn is found in woods, thickets, hedges, and other places throughout the temperate zones of the Northern Hemisphere. It is frequently cultivated.

PLANT DESCRIPTION

It is a thorny shrub or small tree growing to a height of about 5–6 m (20 ft). The leaves are lobed and obovate; the flowers are white, giving rise to red, egg-shaped fruits (haws). Chinese haw is *C. pinnatifida*.

Extracts of fruits, leaves, and flowers are used in herbal medicine.

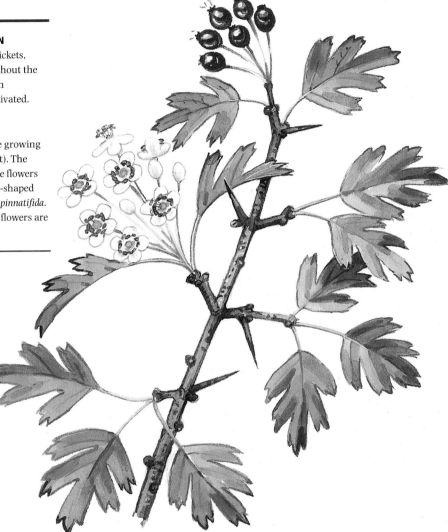

CULINARY AND NUTRITIONAL VALUE

Fruits have been candied and made into jam, jelly, or wine.

CLAIMS AND FOLKLORE

Hawthorn extracts have been used as a diuretic, and for their astringent and antispasmodic properties, but their main application has been for problems of the heart and circulatory system, such as angina, atherosclerosis, and ischaemia. They are also said to increase cardiac perform-ance, and to decrease peripheral vascular resistance, blood pressure, and blood lipids.

EVIDENCE

Among the chemical substances present in hawthorn, the flavonoids have been suggested as the active principles involved in its herbal actions. Human and animal studies have given support to its claimed efficacy, although there is scope for further research. Under certain conditions, there is support for hawthorn as a herbal drug in Germany; the leaf with flower is accepted, but not leaf, flower, and fruit separately.

Because of its action on the heart and circulatory system, self-treatment should be avoided – professional advice is required. Also, hawthorn should not be taken during pregnancy and lactation.

Helonias, false unicorn
Chamaelirium luteum syn. Helonias dioica

Family Liliaceae

ORIGIN AND CULTIVATION
Helonias is found growing wild in eastern North America. It is rarely cultivated. The plant was used by native North Americans, and then adopted by the settlers in the eighteenth and nineteenth centuries.

PLANT DESCRIPTION
The plant is an herbaceous perennial growing to a height of 1 m (3 ft), with a basal rosette of obovate to spoon-shaped leaves, up to 20 cm (8 in) in length. Its flowering stem is erect, and bears small leaves and a dense raceme of tiny green–white flowers. Helonias plants are male or female.

Its root is the source of the herbal drug.

CULINARY AND NUTRITIONAL VALUE
None.

CLAIMS AND FOLKLORE
Helonias has been used mainly to treat gynaecological problems such as menstrual and menopausal complaints, endometriosis, fibroids, threatened miscarriage, and morning sickness, but also as a diuretic, and to expel intestinal worms.

EVIDENCE
Limited chemical information is available, but it is said to contain a steroidal saponin glycoside and another glycoside.

There appears to be no scientific evidence to support its herbal use and, in addition, no data on its toxicity. Consequently it is best avoided, although some modern herbalists are enthusiastic about its use.

Hemp seed *Cannabis sativa*

Family Cannabaceae

ORIGIN AND CULTIVATION

Hemp originated in central Asia and is one of the oldest cultivated crops. During a very early period it was grown in the principal Asiatic countries, and was taken to Europe centuries before the Christian era.

It has been cultivated for three separate purposes: oilseeds, fibre, and narcotic drugs, e.g. 'marijuana'. Cultivation takes place in a number of countries: Russia, Manchuria, China, France, Canada, and others. Plants grown for oil and fibre are often varieties (cultivars) with a very low content of narcotic principles (cannabinoids). In some countries there are legal restrictions.

The seed or seed oil is now sometimes available in health food stores and similar outlets. Before processing, seed is cleaned because of impurities, such as resin, remaining from the plants. Seed itself contains very little or no cannabinoids. In the USA seed is steam or heat sterilized to prevent further germination.

PLANT DESCRIPTION

Hemp seed (botanically, a fruit) is up to 5 mm ($\frac{1}{5}$ in) long and 3 mm ($\frac{1}{8}$ in) broad. It is brown in colour and marked with delicate white veins. The seed is an oval, somewhat flattened structure with two ribs, one on each of the narrow sides. The hemp plant is an annual herb growing to a height of 1–4 m (13 ft). Plants are either male or female.

CULINARY AND NUTRITIONAL VALUE

The seed has been utilized as a food in a number of countries; e.g. in China it is toasted and sold like popcorn, and in Japan it is used as a condiment. Its flour can be mixed with any flour to produce bread, cakes, pastas, and cookies.

Extracted oil has been added to salad dressings and dips. It is not suitable for frying, although it can tolerate short periods of moderate heat. The oil is included in cosmetics and can be used for massage.

The seed contains 30% oil, 20% protein, 35% carbohydrate, and 500 kcal per 100 g. Its oil is unsaturated with a good ratio of the essential fatty acids – linoleic and linolenic. The protein is made up of all the essential amino acids and is said to be very easy to digest. Vitamins present include carotene (precursor to vitamin A), vitamin E, and B vitamins. Some reports have claimed the presence of vitamin C and minute amounts of vitamin D (rather

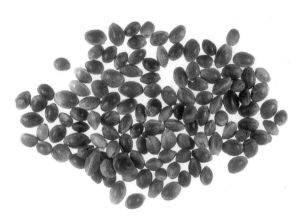

unlikely). There are good amounts of calcium, magnesium, phosphorus, potassium, and sulphur. It supplies dietary fibre (mainly insoluble).

Henna *Lawsonia inermis syn. L. alba*

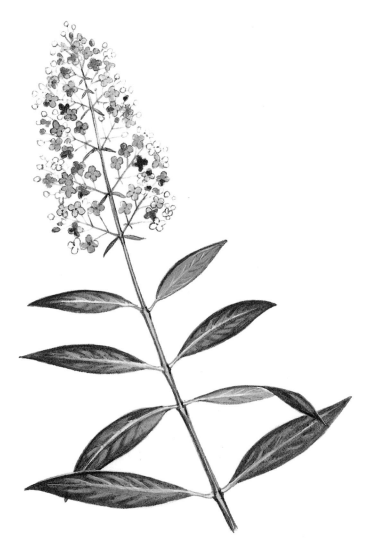

Family Lythraceae

ORIGIN AND CULTIVATION

Henna is an evergreen shrub, considered native to Africa and Asia but also naturalized in America and Australia. It is widely cultivated in tropical regions, e.g. Egypt, Sudan, China, India, Florida, and the West Indies.

Although the plant has had some herbal uses, it is best known as a source of an orange–red dye, obtained from the leaves. It has been used in the Middle East, Far East, and North Africa since ancient times as a colouring for hair, skin, nails, hands, and clothing. Henna was introduced to Europe at the end of the nineteenth century, and became an important constituent of hair tints and conditioners. It is said to fade naturally and does not harm the hair or scalp. Henna can be mixed with other dyes (possibly of plant origin) to give different shades.

A lilac-scented oil obtained from the plant has been used in perfumery. Traditionally, it has been planted as a windbreak for vineyards.

PLANT DESCRIPTION

Henna grows to a height of about 6 m (20 ft), with oblong-shaped leaves up to 5 cm (2 in) in length. The small white to pink highly scented flowers are in clusters and give rise to blue–black capsules.

CULINARY AND NUTRITIONAL VALUE

None.

CLAIMS AND FOLKLORE

Henna has been used mainly in Ayurvedic medicine. It is said to be antibacterial, and is given externally for various skin diseases (including leprosy). Internally, henna has been used to treat diarrhoea and dysentery.

EVIDENCE

It has been stated that lawsone (a naphthoquinone, 0.55–1.0%) is the major active principle, both in colouring and herbal treatment. No clinical or scientific investigations have been found in the literature.

Holy thistle, blessed thistle *Cnicus benedictus*

Family Compositae/Asteraceae

ORIGIN AND CULTIVATION

Holy thistle originated in the Mediterranean region and became naturalized in central and southeastern Europe, and in the eastern USA. It grows in waste places and fields.

PLANT DESCRIPTION

The plant is an annual with bristly branched stems; the white-veined leaves have wavy margins, and lobes ending in sharp spines. Its flower heads are up to 4 cm ($1\frac{1}{2}$ in) across, and consist of yellow florets enclosed in bristly bracts. Holy thistle grows to a height of 65 cm (2 ft).

The aerial parts, including the flower heads are used to make the herbal drug.

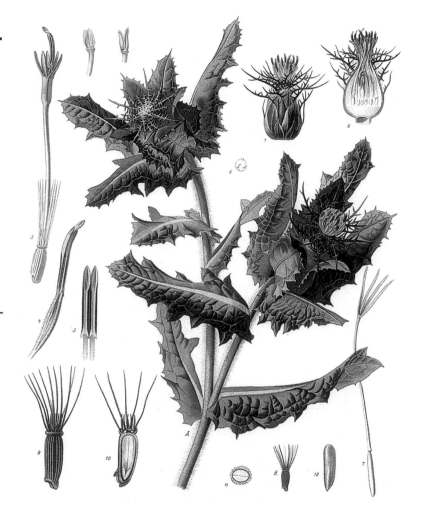

CULINARY AND NUTRITIONAL VALUE

Extracts are included in the liqueur Benedictine, and bitters.

CLAIMS AND FOLKLORE

Holy thistle has been utilized in herbal medicine since the sixteenth century. It was grown in monastery gardens, often as a 'cure-all', and was thought to be effective against the Great Plague. In herbal medicine the drug has been used externally to treat boils, wounds, and ulcers, and internally as an appetizer, stomachic, and diuretic, and for anorexia, dyspepsia, colds, and fevers.

EVIDENCE

A number of chemical substances have been identified, including lignans and sesquiterpene lactones.

Some animal experiments have been carried out but there appear to be no human studies. In Germany there is support for the herb as a bitter digestive to treat loss of appetite and dyspepsia. It is subject to legal restrictions in some countries. Because of the lack of data concerning toxicity, an excess should not be taken during pregnancy and lactation.

Hops *Humulus lupulus*

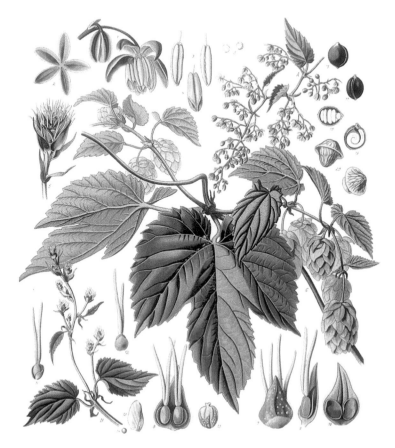

Family Cannabaceae

ORIGIN AND CULTIVATION

The plant is a native of northern Europe, where wild plants can still be found, although it can be difficult to distinguish these from hops that have escaped from cultivation. As it is so important in beer manufacture, cultivation takes place in many countries, e.g. Europe, America, New Zealand, and Australia.

PLANT DESCRIPTION

The crop is a climber that may grow to a height of 6 m (20 ft), and bears leaves usually divided into three or five lobes. Plants are male or female, but the males are normally eliminated to avoid seed set. The female 'cone', the part used in brewing, consists of a cluster of pale yellowish green reduced leaves (bracts and bracteoles) containing the female flowers. Glistening lupulin glands are found on the cone.

CULINARY AND NUTRITIONAL VALUE

Hops were introduced into Britain in the sixteenth century for the purpose of flavouring in beer manufacture. Before that various bitter herbs were used. The lupulin glands produce bitter resins (3–12%) and essential oils (0.3–1%), which contribute to the flavour of beer and, because they are antiseptic, extend its shelf-life.

Extracts and oil of hops are used to flavour various food products, e.g. non-alcoholic beverages, dairy desserts, and confectionery.

The young shoots can be eaten raw or cooked.

CLAIMS AND FOLKLORE

Hops were well established in European medicine by the seventeenth century. The herb (the female 'cone') is taken as a sedative to relieve stress, anxiety, tension, headaches, as an aid to digestion, and for its antispasmodic effect for certain types of asthma and period pains. It is also claimed to alleviate premature ejaculation. Externally, it has been applied for skin infections, eczema, herpes, and leg ulcers.

Commercial preparations often have other herbs added; e.g. as a sedative, valerian is added; for nervous digestive problems, chamomile or peppermint is added.

Dried hops have been included in so-called 'dream' pillows to aid sleep.

EVIDENCE

The herb has been well investigated chemically and a large number of constituents identified. Of these the resins or oleoresins (e.g. humulone and lupulone) and essential oils have been considered the principal active constituents.

Hops (sometimes with the addition of other herbs) have been the subject of a number of animal and human investigations. The herb has some antibacterial activity that might be of importance in its external uses. There is also support for its reputed sedative and antispasmodic activities.

It should not be given to patients suffering from depression or to women during pregnancy and lactation.

The herb is supported in Germany.

Horsetail *Equisetum arvense*

Family Equisetaceae

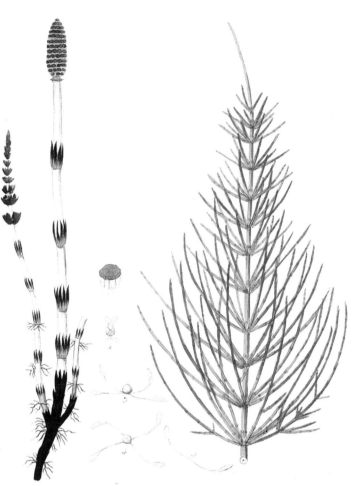

ORIGIN AND CULTIVATION
The horsetail species are found in most temperate regions of the world except Australasia. They reproduce by spores, not by seeds as is normal in herbal plants. Horsetails are a remnant group; they were at their peak some 300 million years ago (the Palaeozoic era) when so-called giant forms existed. They are rich in silica, and because of their abrasive properties were used at one time to scour pots and pans, especially pewter ones.

PLANT DESCRIPTION
At the beginning of the growing season the first structures to appear above ground are pinkish stems up to about 20 cm (8 in) in height, bearing cones with the spores at their tips. After these die down they are replaced by green stems up to about 80 cm (30 in) in height, which are jointed with black-toothed sheaths (reduced leaves) at the nodes and whorls of spreading green branches.

   Equisetum arvense found in fields, and waste or moist places, is the usual species utilized in herbal medicine.

CULINARY AND NUTRITIONAL VALUE
None.

CLAIMS AND FOLKLORE
Horsetail is said to have diuretic and astringent properties. It is claimed to be an excellent clotting agent, with external use in wound healing and curing nose bleeds. Internally it is thought to have a beneficial effect regarding conditions of the genitourinary system, such as cystitis, urethritis, and prostate disease.

   Other claims have been made regarding the efficacy of horsetail, e.g. that the herb added to a bath helps slow-healing sprains and fractures, and skin conditions such as eczema. It was also once used for lung problems, as an anti-tuberculosis drug.

   A French patent exists for the use of isolated silica compounds in the treatment of bone fractures and osteoporosis.

In Canada, manufacturers are required to prove that *E. arvense* products are free of thiaminase-like (enzyme) activity. There is worry that thiamin (vitamin B_1) in the body might be reduced, leading to a deficiency that could affect the brain.

EVIDENCE
Of the substances present in horsetail, silicic acid and silicates are present in large amounts (about 15%). There are also alkaloids, including nicotine (a tiny amount). Some writers relate the therapeutic value of *Equisetum* to silicic acid and silicates.

   Horsetail should not be used for more than 6 weeks. Also the herb should not be given to those with impaired heart or kidney function.

   No scientific studies have been identified that endorse the herbal use of horsetail, but there is support for the plant in Germany.

Hyssop *Hyssopus officinalis*

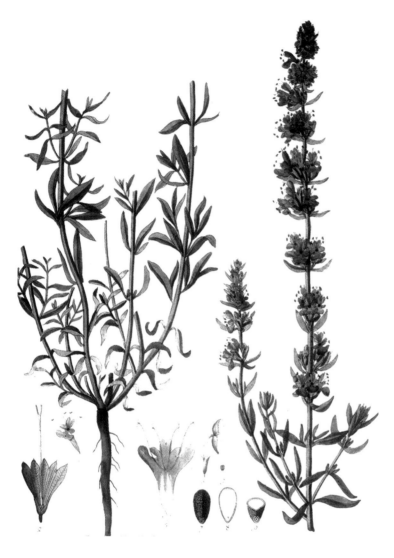

Family Labiatae/Lamiaceae

ORIGIN AND CULTIVATION
Hyssop is native to central and southern Europe, western Asia, and North Africa. It is naturalized in the USA. Major producing countries include France, Hungary, and Holland.

PLANT DESCRIPTION
The herb is a semi-evergreen perennial, woody at the base, with linear leaves up to 2.5 cm (1 in) in length, and growing to a height of 45–60 cm (2 ft). Spikes of two-lipped tubular purple–blue flowers are produced.

The parts used are the leaves and flowering tops. Hyssop essential oil is obtained by steam distillation.

CULINARY AND NUTRITIONAL VALUE
Hyssop extracts and oil may be found in bitters and liqueurs (e.g. Benedictine and chartreuse), non-alcoholic beverages, pickles, meat dishes, confectionery, baked goods, and other food products. The leaves have a somewhat bitter flavour so it should be used sparingly. The oil is a fragrance component in soaps, creams, lotions, and perfumes.

CLAIMS AND FOLKLORE
In early times, because of its scent, hyssop was used in the home to 'cleanse' the air. As a herbal medicine it is used as an expectorant and for various chest problems (e.g. coughs, catarrh, bronchitis). It may also soothe the digestive tract.

EVIDENCE
Apart from a number of other constituents, hyssop produces an essential oil (0.3–2%) that contains, among other substances, camphor. No scientific evidence has been found that supports its therapeutic use and, for this reason, it is not recommended in Germany, although the herb can be used below 5% in tea mixtures.

Care should be taken in using the essential oil as a herbal medicine, because it can induce epileptic seizures and is subject to legal restrictions in some countries.

Ipecacuanha *Cephaelis ipecacuanha*

Family Rubiaceae

ORIGIN AND CULTIVATION

Ipecacuanha was known to the native Brazilians for centuries before being introduced to Portugal in colonial times. Some cultivation has also taken place in Singapore and Malaysia.

PLANT DESCRIPTION

The herb is a shrub growing to a height of 30 cm (1 ft), with oblong pointed leaves. Its small white flowers give rise to purple–black berries.

Roots are the source of the herbal drug.

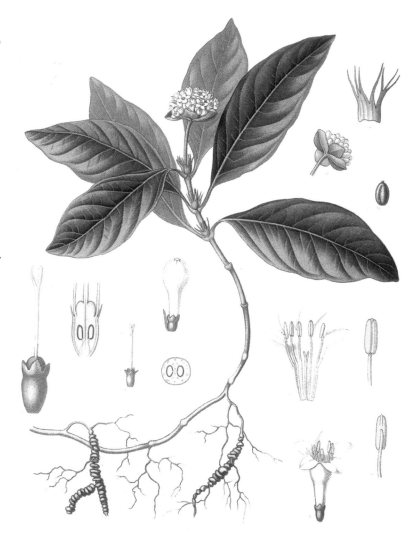

CULINARY AND NUTRITIONAL VALUE

None.

CLAIMS AND FOLKLORE

Ipecacuanha is an expectorant, and found in mixtures for coughs, bronchitis, and whooping cough. At larger doses it acts as an emetic, causing vomiting and diarrhoea. It has therefore been used for drug and poison overdoses. Extracts have been used for amoebic (not bacillary) dysentery.

EVIDENCE

The active principles are alkaloids (isoquinoline), including emetine and cephoeline. Other substances present include tannins and glycosides.

Care should be taken with ipecacuanha. In cough mixtures, the recommended dosages should be followed carefully. Even greater care is required when it is used as an emetic. It should not be given to children when the swallowed poisons are substances such as alkalis, strong acids, strychnine, and cleaning fluids. There have been a number of fatalities in cases where too much ipecacuanha has been used.

Jojoba *Simmondsia chinensis syn. S. californica*

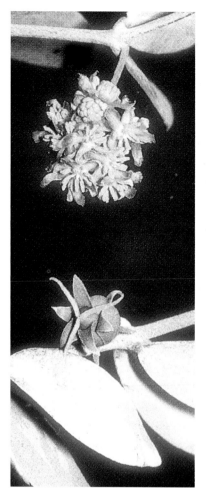

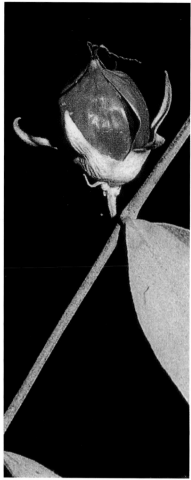

Family Buxaceae

ORIGIN AND CULTIVATION
Jojoba is native to the southwestern USA and Mexico and is found in arid habitats, normally below 1 500 m (5000 ft). It is now cultivated in different parts of the world (e.g. Arizona and the Middle East) for pharmaceutical industries, erosion control, and desert reclamation. The bushes are male or female and distinction can only be made after 3 years. Jojoba is slow growing but tissue culture of female plants has greatly increased production.

PLANT DESCRIPTION
The plant, with thick leathery leaves 2–4 cm ($1\frac{1}{2}$ in) in length, is an evergreen, much-branched shrub, 1–2 m (7 ft) in height with a spread of 1–2 m. In the spring, the male bush produces small yellow flowers in clusters; the female has solitary pale green flowers that give rise to dark brown nut-like fruits, each containing a single seed, 1.5–2 cm ($\frac{4}{5}$ in) in length.

Male flowers.

Female flower.

CULINARY AND NUTRITIONAL VALUE
The seeds have long been known as a source of food to North American Indians, and have been roasted or dried, and then ground and mixed with sugar and water to give a beverage.

CLAIMS AND FOLKLORE
The seed oil has been extracted by the local North American Indians and used in medicine and as a hair restorer.

This oil is not a normal plant oil (triglyceride) but, in fact, a liquid wax. It is an excellent substitute for sperm whale oil, which is good news for whale conservation. Consequently, the oil is found in a wide range of cosmetics (e.g. shampoos, moisturizers, sunscreens), and applied externally for dry skin, psoriasis, acne, and sunburn. It would also make a good industrial lubricant but is really too expensive for that purpose.

EVIDENCE
As far as can be established, there is little experimental evidence to support the use of jojoba oil in treating medical conditions of the skin.

Kava kava *Piper methysticum*

Family Piperaceac

ORIGIN AND CULTIVATION

Kava kava is a plant that plays an important part in the traditional life of the peoples of the tropical South Pacific islands where it is cultivated; it is also cultivated in the USA and Australia. The plant may have evolved from *Piper wichmannii*.

PLANT DESCRIPTION

It is a shrub growing to a height of 3 m (10 ft), with large leaves up to 25 cm (10 in) across. The small flowers are in spikes.

The part of the plant producing a drink and herbal medicine is the rootstock, probably an upright rhizome.

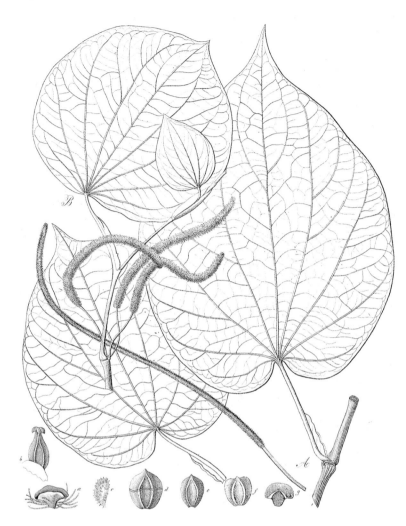

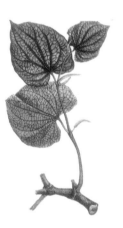

CULINARY AND NUTRITIONAL VALUE

From the kava kava rootstock is produced a beverage that is consumed during various rituals or ceremonies – these have sometimes been likened to wine-drinking social gatherings in Western society. Kava kava beverage stimulates and relaxes the consumer, although heavy consumption can lead to prostration and unconsciousness. Also, prolonged use of kava kava can produce unpleasant symptoms such as skin yellowing and redness of the eyes.

CLAIMS AND FOLKLORE

Extracts are claimed to have certain therapeutic qualities, e.g. that it acts as a diuretic, an analgesic, a urinary antiseptic, and a sedative. The best known modern use is for reducing nervous anxiety and tension.

EVIDENCE

The rootstock contains various chemical substances, such as starch, sugars, and 3–20% kava lactones (resin), presumably the active principles.

Clinical studies and experience, particularly in Germany, have led to the conclusion that kava kava products can be effective at dealing with mild states of anxiety, and are a reasonable alternative to synthetic tranquillizers such as benzodiazepines.

Consumption of kava kava as a herbal may lead to the same side-effects as described under its use as a beverage; also, it should not be consumed with alcohol, and, if consumed machinery should not be worked.

Kava kava must not be used during pregnancy and lactation. The drug has been removed from sale in the UK.

Lavender *Lavandula species*

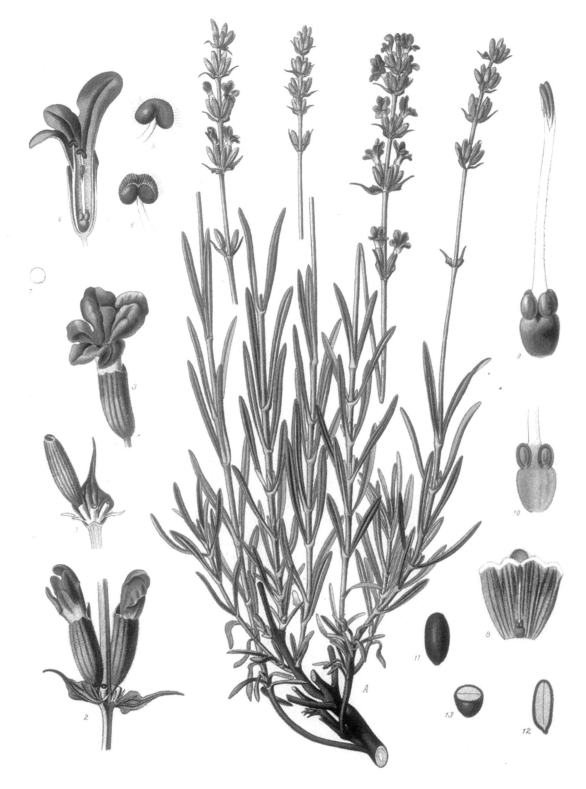

Lavender

Family Labiatae/Lamiaceae

ORIGIN AND CULTIVATION

The various lavender species are grown for their flowers and essential oil. True or garden lavender (*Lavandula angustifolia* syn. *L. officinalis*) is a native of the northern Mediterranean region, but is now cultivated in other countries – France is well known in this connection. Broad-leaved lavender (*L. latifolia*) is also a native of the Mediterranean region and is cultivated. Lavandin (*L. × intermedia*) is a hybrid of *angustifolia* and *latifolia*, and is cultivated.

The oil obtained by steam distillation from *L. angustifolia* is used in perfumes, colognes, and toilet articles. That from *L. latifolia* and *L. × intermedia* has a rather pungent and camphoraceous odour, and is used mainly in cleaning products and insect repellents.

Other lavender species of economic importance include *L. stoechas* and *L. allardii*.

PLANT DESCRIPTION

- *L. angustifolia* is an evergreen sub-shrub, with woody stems attaining a length of 20–30 cm (1 ft) and covered in small linear leaves. The small, blue, two-lipped flowers are carried on leafless stems, which grow above the leaves to a height of about 60 cm (2 ft).

- *L. latifolia* differs from *L. angustifolia* in a number of respects; e.g. the plant is larger and the leaves are spoon shaped, not linear.

- *L. × intermedia* is intermediate in character between the two previous species.

CULINARY AND NUTRITIONAL VALUE

Flowers may be crystallized or added to jams, ice-cream, confectionery, and other foods.

CLAIMS AND FOLKLORE

Lavender has been known as a herbal medicine since the late Middle Ages, and was taken to North America by the Pilgrim Fathers in the early seventeenth century.

Extracts of the flower have been taken internally or applied externally. Taken internally, they were said to be good for indigestion, relaxing spasms, and stimulating peripheral circulation, and to act against depression, anxiety, exhaustion, and similar complaints. The oil is antiseptic and antibacterial, and can be applied externally for headaches, burns, sunburn, neuralgia, and other conditions.

The oil may be added to a bath for relaxation purposes or used in aromatherapy.

EVIDENCE

The essential oil (0.5–1.5%), with over 100 components, seems to be an important therapeutic substance, although it should not be taken internally unless under professional supervision.

There has been recent interest in the external application of the oil (including in aromatherapy) as a sedative, tranquillizer, and treatment for insomnia. A small number of clinical trials have been carried out, which support the previous claims. The oil is non-toxic and is supported in Germany.

Lecithin

ORIGIN
Lecithin is a phospholipid – a combination of phosphorus and fatty substances. It is a common compound in the cells of all living organisms and is required for proper biological functioning. The best known commercial source is the soya bean, but it has also been extracted from eggs and brains.

CULINARY AND NUTRITIONAL VALUE
In the food industry, lecithin is well known as an emulsifier and stabilizer in the manufacture of margarine (margarine is an emulsion of water in oil). It is also used in the production of other items such as confectionery, snack foods, baked goods, cheese, meat, poultry, and dairy products.

It first became available commercially during the 1930s.

CLAIMS AND FOLKLORE
Lecithin, it has been claimed, reduces blood cholesterol, controls or prevents atherosclerosis, and is an effective treatment for dementia, Alzheimer's disease, and various liver disorders (e.g. hepatitis, cirrhosis, toxic damage).

EVIDENCE
There is some scientific evidence that lecithin is an agent in reducing blood cholesterol and a valid treatment for liver disorders but, as yet, there is no support for the other claims. It has no use as a slimming agent, although there have been suggestions to the contrary.

Lecithin has a low toxicity but is not recommended for use during pregnancy. It is recognized in Germany for some functions.

Lime flower, linden flower *Tilia species*

Family Tiliaceae

ORIGIN AND CULTIVATION

The flowers of a number of *Tilia* species are utilized in herbal medicine, e.g. *T. cordata*, *T. platyphyllos*, *T. × europaea* (a hybrid of the two previous species), and *T. americana*. Lime is found wild in Europe but is also extensively cultivated in parks and similar places.

PLANT DESCRIPTION

Lime is a large tree, growing to a height of 10–30 m (100 ft), with shiny, heart-shaped leaves. It produces yellow–white flowers that give rise to round green fruits.

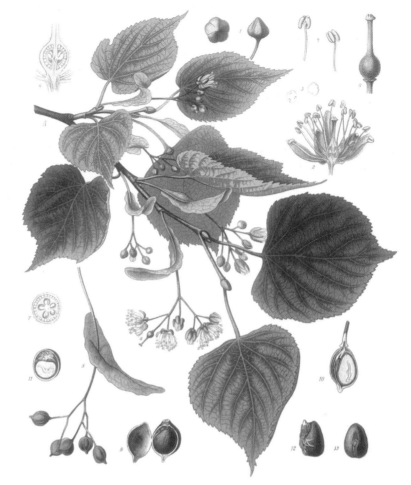

CULINARY AND NUTRITIONAL VALUE

Lime or linden flowers can be found in teas and honey.

CLAIMS AND FOLKLORE

A number of therapeutic claims have been made for the flowers. They are said to have a sedative or tranquillizing effect, and are therefore useful in dealing with cardiovascular (e.g. high blood pressure) and digestive problems associated with anxiety. Similarly, they might assist with migraines and headaches. The flowers increase the rate of sweating and consequently can be useful with feverish colds, influenza, and respiratory catarrh. Other claims relate to the herb being antispasmodic and acting as a diuretic. Lime flower extracts have been included in lotions for itchy skin.

EVIDENCE

The chemistry of lime flower has been well investigated. Few scientific investigations seem to have been carried out into its efficacy, although some animal studies support its antispasmodic property. Usually this activity and its value in increasing the rate of sweating are related to the flavonoids and p-coumaric acid present. Essential oils have also been implicated in some of the effects, including the sedative action of lime flower.

Excessive use of the herb should be avoided, not just in pregnancy and lactation, but generally, because there is a possibility that it may cause cardiac damage.

Some support is given to the herb in Germany.

Linseed, flax *Linum usitatissimum*

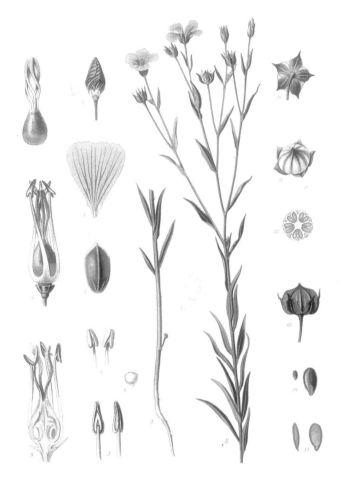

Family Linaceae

ORIGIN AND CULTIVATION
Linseed is one of the oldest crops known to the human species; it has been cultivated for at least 7000 years. The plant probably evolved in the Mediterranean area, possibly from the wild species *Linum angustifolia* or *L. perenne*. It is now grown in many parts of the world, and is somewhat unusual in that one form provides seed and seed oil, while another produces stem fibre (flax).

PLANT DESCRIPTION
The plant is an annual herb growing to a height of 80–160 cm (5 ft). The leaves are pointed and the flowers bright blue (white in some forms). Its fruits are capsules containing oval, flattened, pale to dark brown shiny seeds 4–6 mm ($\frac{1}{4}$ in) in length.

CULINARY AND NUTRITIONAL VALUE
The seed contains 30–40% oil (mainly linoleic and linolenic acids) and about 25% protein. It and the residue after oil extraction are well known livestock feeds. The oil is a drying oil, and consequently used in the manufacture of paints, varnishes, and linoleum. In some parts of the world it has been utilized for human food.

Seeds are available in health food shops.

CLAIMS AND FOLKLORE
Taken internally the seeds act as a bulk laxative (due in part, at least, to the copious mucilage produced by the skin of the seed). It has also been claimed that linseed taken internally assists with gastritis, pharyngitis, chronic bronchial complaints, coughs, sore throat, eczema, and other problems.

Applied externally as a poultice, linseed is claimed to ease bronchitis, pleurisy, burns, and boils.

EVIDENCE
The results of only very few scientific investigations seem to be available concerning the efficacy of linseed. Some preliminary experiments with humans indicate that linseed in the diet reduces total blood cholesterol in hypercholesterolaemic patients. Clearly more work is required.

It has been known for a long time that linseed contains a cyanogenic glycoside known as linamarin, which under certain conditions produces toxic prussic acid. To avoid this problem, the seed has often been boiled prior to inclusion in animal feed. As regards human food, the same practice could well be followed. It has also been suggested that young seeds should be avoided and doses carefully adhered to.

Support is given to the use of the seed in Germany.

Liquorice *Glycyrrhiza glabra*

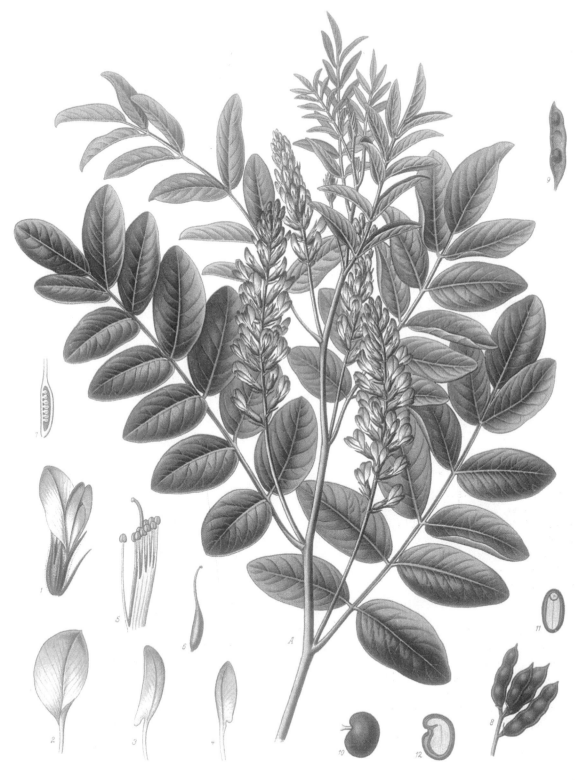

Liquorice

Family Leguminosae/Fabaceae

ORIGIN AND CULTIVATION

It grows wild throughout southern Europe, Russia, the Middle East, and Afghanistan. Today the main cultivation takes place in Spain, Italy, Russia, and Turkey.

Glycyrrhiza lepidota (American or wild liquorice) was used by the native North Americans and early settlers for problems with childbirth and menstruation, and *G. uralensis* was known in traditional Chinese medicine. However, *G. glabra* is the usual liquorice. The root and stolons are utilized.

PLANT DESCRIPTION

Liquorice is a perennial herb that grows to a height of just over 1 m (3 ft). Its pinnate leaves are composed of 9–17 leaflets. The numerous blue flowers, 1–1.5 cm ($\frac{3}{5}$ in) in length, are borne in long conical heads; they give rise to reddish brown pods 1.5–2.5 cm (1 in) in length, which contain three or four seeds. Under cultivation, the crop is allowed to grow for 3–5 years before being harvested, by which time it will have formed an extensive system of roots and stolons, which, in well drained soils, may reach a depth of about 1 m (3 ft) and a spread of several metres.

CULINARY AND NUTRITIONAL VALUE

The root contains the glycoside glycyrrhizin, which is 50 times sweeter than sucrose sugar. It is possible that the dried root is still sold as confectionery, but usually the juice is obtained from the root and concentrated by boiling. The solid extract thus obtained is found as liquorice sticks, and in candy and chewing gum. Extracts are used to flavour tobacco, beer, soft drinks, frozen dairy desserts, and baked goods.

CLAIMS AND FOLKLORE

Liquorice was an important medical herb in ancient Egypt, Assyria, China, Greece, and no doubt other countries. It did not reach Europe until the fifteenth century. The plant was introduced by Dominican friars to Pontefract, Yorkshire, UK, which became famous for the production of Pontefract cakes or pomfreys (liquorice lozenges).

Extracts are used in cough drops, syrups, tonics, laxatives, antismoking lozenges, tea, capsules, tinctures, and tablets, and it is said to have demulcent, expectorant, antitussive, anti-inflammatory, and mild laxative properties. Liquorice has been used to treat bronchial catarrh, bronchitis, arthritis, inflamed joints, some skin problems, inflammatory conditions of the digestive system (e.g. mouth ulcers, gastritis, peptic ulcers), and as a flavouring to mask undesirable tastes in medicine, e.g. cascara.

EVIDENCE

Analyses have revealed a wide range of chemical constituents, the best known being the glycoside glycyrrhizin. On the whole, animal and human studies have supported the traditional uses of liquorice. It is approved in Germany. However, excessive use of the material should be avoided, because this can raise blood pressure and lead to water retention in those already exhibiting high blood pressure or kidney disease, or taking digoxin-based medication. It is best avoided by pregnant women.

Lobelia, Indian tobacco *Lobelia inflata*

Family Campanulaceae

ORIGIN AND CULTIVATION
Lobelia inflata is native to parts of North America, growing in neglected areas and by roadsides. Other species that have been used for medicinal purposes are *L. siphilitica*, *L. tupa*, and *L. chinensis*.

PLANT DESCRIPTION
The plant is a hairy annual, growing to a height of 1 m (3 ft) and with ovate, toothed leaves 5–8 cm (3 in) in length. Its pale blue, pink-tinged flowers give rise to two-valved capsules.

The aerial parts (stem and leaves) are used in herbal medicine.

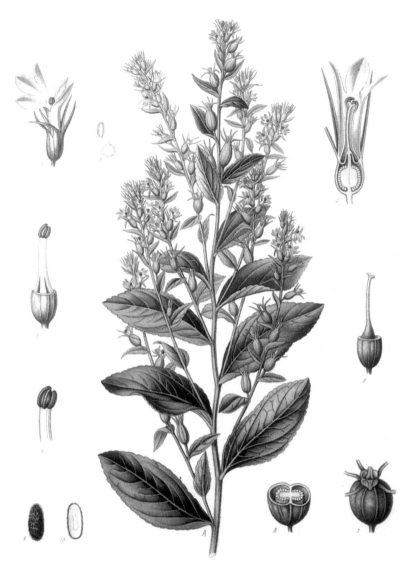

CULINARY AND NUTRITIONAL VALUE
None.

CLAIMS AND FOLKLORE
Native North Americans and settlers used lobelia for a variety of purposes: to relieve asthma, and to treat dysentery, epilepsy, diphtheria, and whooping cough. Some modern herbalists use its strong antispasmodic properties to treat asthma and bronchitis, and employ it externally for sprains and back problems.

EVIDENCE
The active principles are alkaloids, particularly lobeline.

Too much lobelia can lead to convulsions and collapse. Worry about overdosage has led to some herbalists not using the drug and some manufacturers not including it in their products.

Lobelia has been used in antismoking preparations, although this has not been allowed in the USA since 1993.

Lycopodium, clubmoss *Lycopodium clavatum*

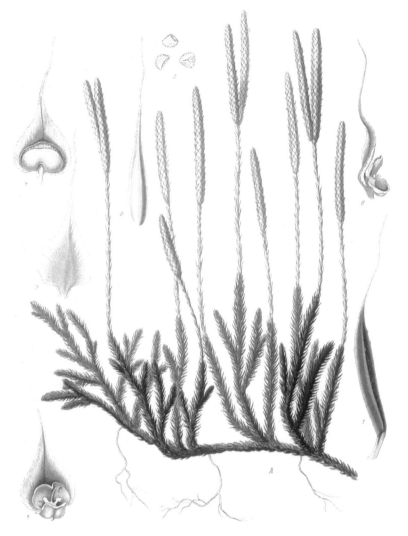

Family Lycopodiaceae

ORIGIN AND CULTIVATION

Lycopodium clavatum (common clubmoss) is found growing on mountains and moorland throughout temperate regions of the Northern Hemisphere. There are other *Lycopodium* species. Like the living horsetails, clubmosses are a remnant group – they reached their peak in the Palaeozoic era (some 300 million years ago) when giant forms existed. Like horsetails, they reproduce by spores, not seeds.

PLANT DESCRIPTION

The common clubmoss has creeping stems, 30–60 cm (2 ft) in length, which are covered with stiff, linear green leaves. Upwardly growing branches bear at their tips cones that produce yellow spores.

CULINARY AND NUTRITIONAL VALUE

None.

CLAIMS AND FOLKLORE

Lycopodium has been employed as a medicinal herb since at least the Middle Ages. Extracts of the whole plant have been used as a diuretic – to try to flush out kidney stones and to treat urinary complaints. The herb has been given for indigestion and gastritis. The spores have been used to treat skin complaints and coat tablets.

EVIDENCE

Clubmoss contains alkaloids, polyphenols, flavonoids, and triterpenes. It has not been possible to locate any experimental work.

Margarines and spreads

Margarines and fat spreads are replacements for butter. Historically, the first margarines were said to be produced after a competition to provide a substitute for butter for the French soldiers in the Napoleonic wars. A chemist, Mege-Mourie, discovered that a substance with the texture of butter could be produced by blending a mixture of fats and oils, and this paved the way for the manipulation of fats and oils to produce a variety of products with potential health benefits. Colouring is added, together with flavours and salt to enhance the taste: in addition vitamins A and D are required to be added, to bring them to a level similar to that found naturally in butter. Margarines may contain animal fats, vegetable oils, or sometimes a mixture of both – the types of oils used will be described in the ingredient list.

Margarines generally have similar fat and energy content to butter, but there are also a variety of spreads that are not called margarines because their composition is different. These include a range of reduced-fat spreads that are presented as lower energy spreads for those who wish to reduce fat or energy intake. Surprisingly, although huge amounts of these spreads and other reduced-fat products are now sold in the UK, Europe, and the USA, the incidence of obesity continues to rise. In the UK the term 'low-fat' can only be used for a spread that has no more than 40 g of fat per 100 g (compared with the 80 g plus per 100 g in butter or margarine).

POLYUNSATURATED AND MONOUNSATURATED SPREADS

The greatest growth in margarine sales was initially due to the production of those high in polyunsaturated fatty acids, based on maize or sunflower oils. Soya margarines have also been produced and have relatively high polyunsaturated fatty acid content. Many studies showed that replacing butter or margarines that have a high saturated fat content with those with a high proportion of polyunsaturated fatty acid resulted in a lowering of blood cholesterol levels; however, there was some concern that levels of 'good', i.e. high-density lipoproteins, also fell, causing some scientists to be concerned that consumption of high levels of polyunsaturated fatty acid would not always be beneficial. In the last few years there has been a shift towards the production of spreads, generally based on olive oil, with a high proportion of monounsaturated fatty acids – thus mimicking the fat distribution of the Mediterranean diet. Consumption of these fats does not seem to lower high-density cholesterol.

SPREADS CONTAINING PLANT STANOLS AND STEROLS

These are the most recent additions to the range of spreads. They are sometimes also referred to as phytostanols and phytosterols (phyto = plant). The sterols include beta-sitosterol, campesterol, and stigmasterol, which occur naturally in plants, while the stanols such as sitostanol and campestanol are more 'saturated' compounds which occur only in small amounts in plants. The stanols used in the spreads are therefore manufactured from plant sterols. These plant stanols and sterols have chemical structures that are very similar to cholesterol and they block the absorption of cholesterol in the gastrointestinal tract. They affect the absorption of cholesterol from foods and, more importantly, also prevent reabsorption of cholesterol made in the body, which is excreted into the gastrointestinal tract in bile. The cholesterol in bile is normally reabsorbed lower down the gut and returned to the liver. Prevention of reabsorption means that the body has to manufacture more cholesterol in the liver and draws on blood cholesterol levels to do this. Blood cholesterol levels then fall.

In the UK there are two ranges of products containing these materials on the market, the Benecol™ range (contains plant stanols), and Pro-Activ™ (a low-fat spread that contains plant sterols). The spreads contain about 8 g of active material per 100 g, and there are also yoghurts, semi-skimmed milks, and cereal bars in the Benecol™ range. Recent research has suggested that the materials work just as well in low-fat products and it is likely that the range of such products containing phytosterols and phytostanols will increase.

Consumption of about 2 g of plant sterol or stanol per day (the equivalent of about 25 g of spread) will lower blood low-density lipoprotein cholesterol (the type of cholesterol that is implicated in atherosclerosis development) by about 9–14% when consumed instead of margarine containing polyunsaturated fats. It has been suggested that if you switch from using butter or a margarine containing more saturated fats the effects would be more marked. Studies have also shown that the effects are greater in older people, although the reasons are not clear as yet. It has been suggested that if everyone in the UK consumed 2 g of plant stanols/sterols per day there would be a reduction in coronary heart disease of about 20–25%; not quite as remarkable as some cholesterol-lowering drugs but still very significant. The products are not recommended for women who are pregnant or breast-feeding, or for children under the age of 5 years.

Marigold *Calendula officinalis*

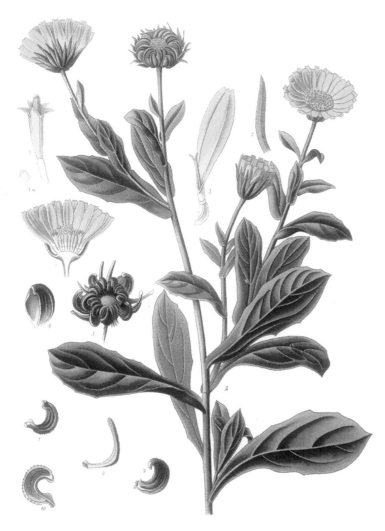

Family Compositae/Asteraceae

ORIGIN AND CULTIVATION
Marigold is possibly a native of southern Europe but is now widely cultivated throughout Europe and North America as an ornamental, medicinal, and culinary plant. It should not be confused with *Tagetes*, also known as marigold.

PLANT DESCRIPTION
The plant is an annual with a branched stem and lanceolate leaves, growing to a height of 50–70 cm (28 in). Yellow to orange florets constitute the flower head, up to 7 cm (3 in) across.

The flower heads are the parts used for culinary and medical purposes.

CULINARY AND NUTRITIONAL VALUE
Marigold petals may be utilized as a substitute for saffron (*Crocus sativus*) in rice and soup, and also included in salads. Extracts of the petals have been used to colour cheese, butter, and other foods.

CLAIMS AND FOLKLORE
Petal extracts, applied externally, have been considered effective in dealing with various skin complaints such as burns, sunburn, inflammation, hard-to-heal wounds, and others. The drug is said to be antiseptic (antibacterial, antiviral, antiparasitic). It is also thought to act as an immunostimulant for skin inflammation and various infections. Marigold is included in skin care products such as ointments, lotions, and shampoos.

The herb has also been used internally for disorders of the alimentary canal such as ulcers, colitis, and diverticulitis.

Marigold has been used internally and externally in homeopathy for injuries where the skin is broken.

EVIDENCE
A number of animal experiments have investigated the efficacy of marigold. Its reputed antiseptic and anti-inflammatory properties have found support; flavonoids and triterpenoids may contribute to the anti-inflammatory effect. The immunostimulant activity has been attributed to polysaccharides.

Marigold is said to be generally non-toxic, although it is best avoided during pregnancy and lactation.

It is approved in Germany.

Marshmallow *Althaea officinalis*

Family Malvaceae

ORIGIN AND CULTIVATION
Marshmallow grows in damp meadows, marshes, estuaries, and salt marshes. It is found in Europe, central Asia, and North Africa, and is also naturalized in the eastern USA.

PLANT DESCRIPTION
The herb is a perennial growing to a height of some 2 m (6 ft). Its upright stem is covered with soft hairs, as are the round to ovate leaves, 3–8 cm (3 in) across. The flowers, 2–4 cm ($1\frac{1}{2}$ in) across, are pale pink. There is a fleshy taproot.

Both leaf and root are used in herbal medicine.

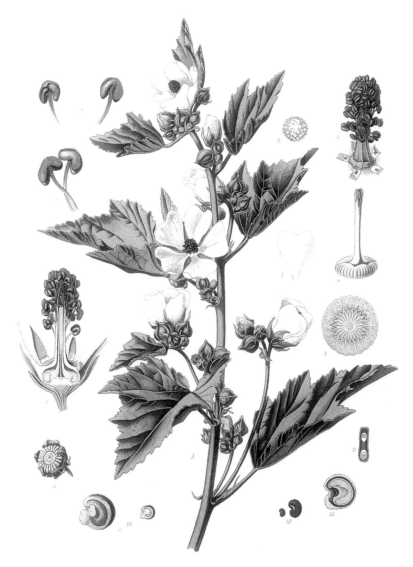

CULINARY AND NUTRITIONAL VALUE
Marshmallow was once included in confectionery.

CLAIMS AND FOLKLORE
The medicinal use of the plant was known to Greek and Arabian physicians some 2000 years ago. Because of its soothing (demulcent) action, marshmallow extract has been taken internally for catarrh, bronchitis, irritating coughs, and problems of the urinary and digestive tract; and externally, for skin disorders such as boils, abscesses, inflammations, and minor injuries.

It may possibly control bacterial infection.

EVIDENCE
The soothing action of marshmallow is related to its mucilage content, 25–35%. One animal study, at least, demonstrated that the plant shows antimicrobial action towards certain bacteria, but there are few experimental investigations on record relating to the efficacy of marshmallow.

Marshmallow is generally non-toxic and is supported in Germany.

Meadowsweet *Filipendula ulmaria*

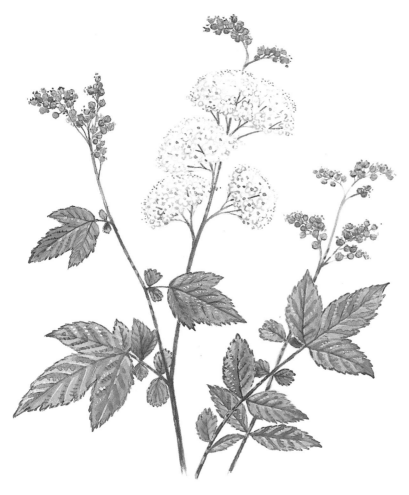

Family Rosaceae

ORIGIN AND CULTIVATION

Meadowsweet grows in moist and marshy soils throughout Europe, temperate Asia, and North America. The plant was one of the sacred herbs of the ancient Druids. In medieval times, and because of its scent, it was a favourite strewing herb. It was from meadowsweet that salicylic acid was first isolated in 1838, and then synthesized in 1889 to give 'aspirin' (named after the old plant name of Spiraea).

PLANT DESCRIPTION

F. ulmaria is a perennial growing up to a height of 1.2 m (4 ft). The leaves, green above and soft whitish below, are pinnately divided. Numerous almond-scented, yellowish white flowers are produced, later giving rise to very small capsules.

The parts utilized in herbal medicine are the flowers and whole plant.

CULINARY AND NUTRITIONAL VALUE

At one time the leaves were added to drinks such as mead, wine, and port.

CLAIMS AND FOLKLORE

Meadowsweet is considered anti-inflammatory and has been used for arthritis and rheumatism. It has been employed for complaints such as acid indigestion, heartburn, and peptic ulcers, and also diarrhoea in children. Unlike the effect of aspirin in certain cases, the herb is said not to upset the stomach lining.

EVIDENCE

Salicylates, flavonoids, and tannins are some of the chemical constituents of meadowsweet. No human studies have been identified, although there is a feeling that the reputed antiseptic, antirheumatic, and astringent actions are justified. No doubt salicylates play an important part. In contrast to certain situations with aspirin, the reported gentle action of meadowsweet on the stomach lining may be the result of an interaction of a number of chemical constituents.

Meadowsweet should not be used by those hypersensitive to aspirin. Although it has been employed as a treatment for diarrhoea in children, this is not recommended – nor is its use during pregnancy and lactation.

In Germany, the drug is approved.

Milk thistle, Mary thistle

Silybum marianum syn. Carduus marianus

Family Compositae/Asteraceae

ORIGIN AND CULTIVATION

Milk thistle probably originated in the Mediterranean region, and is naturalized in much of Europe, North America, South America, and Australia, growing in abandoned fields, old pastures, and by roadsides. It has been cultivated for centuries.

The plant should not be confused with holy thistle (*Cnicus benedictus*).

PLANT DESCRIPTION

Milk thistle can grow to a height of 1.5 m (5 ft) and is an annual or biennial. The leaves have distinctive white markings with spines on the lobes. Its large flower head, surrounded by bracts, consists of purple florets.

The 'seeds' (botanically speaking, the fruits) are the source of herbal medicine.

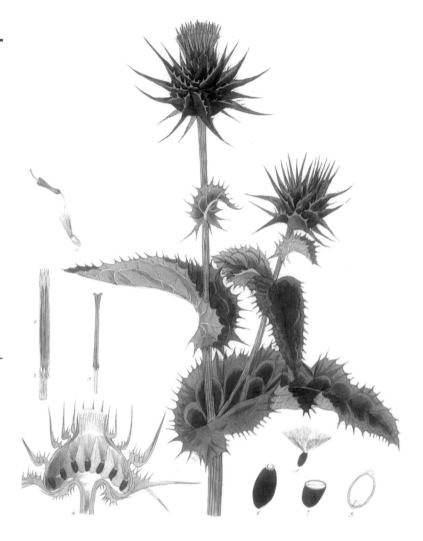

CULINARY AND NUTRITIONAL VALUE

The plant has been utilized as a vegetable and salad item, and the flower receptacle has been used like globe artichoke.

CLAIMS AND FOLKLORE

For hundreds, and maybe thousands, of years it has been used to treat liver disease and damage, including cirrhosis, hepatitis, jaundice, effects of chemotherapy, and poisoning by carbon tetrachloride or amanita mushrooms.

EVIDENCE

A complex known as silymarin (1–4% of which is composed of flavonolignans) is found in the 'seeds'. In Germany, where there has been considerable interest in the drug, it is recommended as a supportive treatment for inflammatory liver conditions and cirrhosis.

For various reasons, it is best given by injection.

Mistletoe *Viscum album*

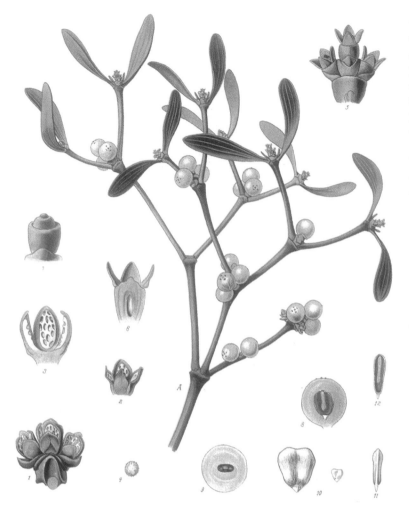

Family Loranthaceae

ORIGIN AND CULTIVATION

Mistletoe is a parasite, growing on trees such as apple, lime, poplar, hawthorn, and rowan, although some may regard the plant as a semiparasite because the leaves contain chlorophyll.

Viscum album is found throughout temperate Europe and extends into Asia. American mistletoe is *Phoradendron leucarpum*.

PLANT DESCRIPTION

It is an evergreen shrub, with regularly branched stems, leathery, oval yellow–green leaves, and up to 3 m (10 ft) across. In the spring, tiny yellow flowers are produced that give rise to sticky, white berries.

CULINARY AND NUTRITIONAL VALUE

All parts of the plant are toxic if eaten.

CLAIMS AND FOLKLORE

Mistletoe was regarded by the ancient Druids as a herb with magical powers. Taken internally, it is claimed that mistletoe extract lowers blood pressure, and is a tonic for the heart, an immunostimulant, an antispasmodic, a sedative, a diuretic, and has certain anticancer effects. Applied externally, it is supposed to be effective against arthritis, rheumatism, chilblains, leg ulcers, and varicose veins.

EVIDENCE

A large number of animal and human studies have looked at the efficacy of mistletoe. They have concentrated on the possible anticancer and immunostimulant properties of the plant. Much is known about the chemical constituents of mistletoe, and because the plant is a parasite it is possible that some of these are taken from the host plant and will vary according to the identity of the host.

The experiments have supported, to some extent, the anticancer and immunostimulant actions of mistletoe. Indeed, there is available a commercial preparation of mistletoe for the treatment of cancer, although it is suggested that this should only be used as an adjunct to conventional practice. Viscotoxins (proteins) in the plant are regarded as the active anticancer agents. The herb is supported in Germany.

Because of potential toxicity, mistletoe should only be used under the guidance of an experienced herbal practitioner, and should be avoided during pregnancy and lactation.

Motherwort *Leonurus cardiaca*

Family Labiatae/Lamiaceae

ORIGIN AND CULTIVATION
It is said to be native to central Asia but is naturalized in Europe and North America, growing in hedges, waste places, and on roadsides. Motherwort is cultivated as a garden plant.

Other related species used in herbal medicine are *Leonurus sibiricus* and *L. heterophyllus*.

PLANT DESCRIPTION
The plant is a perennial growing to 1.5 m (5 ft) in height. Its leaves are divided into five- or seven-toothed lobes. The flowers are pink or white with a very hairy upper lip.

Aerial parts of the plant provide the drug.

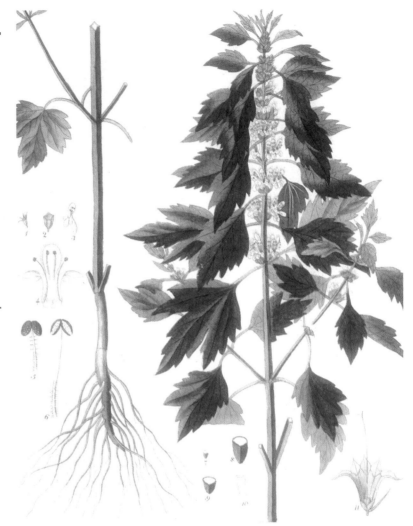

CULINARY OR NUTRITIONAL VALUE
None.

CLAIMS AND FOLKLORE
Motherwort has been used to treat problems of the heart, menstruation, and menopause, especially if they have been considered of nervous origin.

EVIDENCE
The plant contains alkaloids, flavonoids, iridoids, tannins, and other substances. Some animal experiments might support its action on the heart, but self-diagnosis of, and self-medication for, heart problems are considered medically unsuitable. Therefore, herbal medicine from motherwort should be treated very carefully and not used by those on heart medication, or during pregnancy and lactation. The herb is supported in Germany.

Nettle *Urtica dioica*

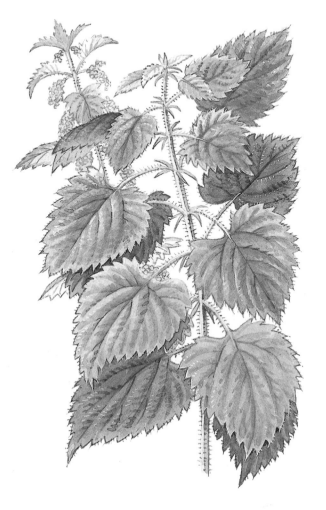

Family Urticaceae

ORIGIN AND CULTIVATION
Nettle is found in waste places, on roadsides, and along hedges throughout Europe, and has been carried as a weed to many other parts of the world, including North America.

PLANT DESCRIPTION
Urtica dioica is a perennial, growing to a height of about 1.5 m (5 ft) and spreading by means of a creeping rhizome. It is well known because of its stinging hairs. The minute green flowers are borne in pendulous clusters, males and females being on separate plants.

 U. urens is the annual nettle, and *U. pilulifera*, the Roman nettle, is said to have been used in the practice of 'urtification', the thrashing of painful arthritic limbs with stems, which acted as a counter-irritant.

 All parts of the plant have been utilized in herbal medicine.

CULINARY AND NUTRITIONAL VALUE
The young plant tops (the older leaves are gritty), gathered when about 15 cm (6 in) high, can be used as a green vegetable, usually in the form of a purée like spinach. Nettles have been processed to make soup, beer, and tea.

 They are rich in vitamin C (75 mg per 100 g) and have high amounts of carotene, iron, calcium, and potassium. There has been commercial extraction of chlorophyll for use as colouring in food and medicines.

CLAIMS AND FOLKLORE
Nettle has been used to treat a number of complaints. Internally, it has been employed as a diuretic and an astringent, to clear toxins, and to reduce blood pressure and blood sugar levels; it has also been used to treat anaemia, haemorrhage (especially of the uterus), excessive menstruation, haemorrhoids, arthritis, rheumatism, gout, and skin complaints (especially eczema). Externally, it has been used to treat arthritic pain, gout, sciatica, neuralgia, haemorrhoids, scalp and hair problems, burns, insect bites, and nose bleeds.

EVIDENCE
There is considerable knowledge concerning the chemical constituents (e.g. glycosides, chlorophyll, vitamins, silicon) of nettle. Clinical studies have investigated the effect of nettle on a number of medical conditions. Some have claimed that urination in men suffering from an enlarged prostate was alleviated. For that reason it (the root) has been used in Germany as supportive treatment for enlarged prostates. Some human studies have indicated a positive value in the treatment of arthritis.

 Nettle should not be used during pregnancy and excessive use should be avoided during lactation.

New Zealand green-lipped mussel *Perna canaliculus*

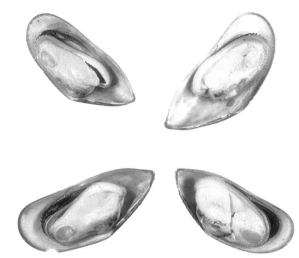

ORIGIN AND CULTIVATION
As the name indicates, the mussel has its origin in New Zealand and is extensively farmed.

CULINARY AND NUTRITIONAL VALUE
The mussel is a well known culinary item and has a nutritional composition of about 14% protein and 2% fat (lipids). Its main mineral elements are sodium, potassium, and phosphorus, with lesser amounts of calcium, magnesium, iron, and some others. Vitamins recorded as present are B_1 (thiamin), B_2 (riboflavin), niacin, and C (ascorbic acid).

CLAIMS AND FOLKLORE
The claimed therapeutic properties of the mussel were a strong impetus for the rapid development of mussel farming in the 1970s in New Zealand. Extracts were said to relieve pain, stiffness, and other symptoms of rheumatoid arthritis and osteoarthritis, with a low incidence of side-effects. It was also claimed that patients showed an improvement in general health. Those who support the claims for the therapeutic value of the mussel extract regard eicosatetraenoic acids as the active principles.

EVIDENCE
Early investigations did provide evidence for the therapeutic value of the mussel extract. However, recent work has not supported this. Therefore, on balance, it is reasonable to assume that the value of mussel extract in treating arthritis is of doubtful significance.

Nutritional supplements

These are supplements, usually ready-made drinks or powders that can be added to milk to make a drink that will replace meals for those who are unable to eat. Some products are also available in the form of soups. Products such as Complan™ and Build-Up™ are sold over the counter. This type of supplement aims to supply all known nutrients for those who cannot eat any food at all, but if consumed in this way they are high-protein drinks. A sick person obtaining 1500 kcal per day would consume about 85 g and 105 g of protein from Build-up and Complan, respectively. If people cannot eat food for more than a day or two advice should be sought from a medical practitioner, who may refer the person to a dietitian.

Other supplements may be available on prescription for people with particular conditions; these are usually prescribed by a doctor on the advice of a dietitian, but may also sometimes be sold over the counter. They may be milk based or fruit based and are ready-made in Tetra Paks. They do not necessarily supply the whole range of nutrients and may therefore not be suitable for people who cannot eat solid food at all.

Table 24 Composition of Build-up and Complan: energy and selected nutrients supplied by a 200 ml portion

	Energy (kcal)	Protein (g)	Fat (g)	CHO[a] (g)	Calcium (mg)	Iron (mg)	Vitamin B_{12} (mg)	Folate (μg)	Vitamin C (mg)	Vitamin D (μg)
Build-up[b]	200	11.2	7.2	23.4	380	2.6	1.4	102	16	2.46
Complan[b]	290	13.8	11.2	33.8	500	3.0	1.6	84	20	1.02
Complan savoury	200	9.8	7.0	24.4	136	2.8	1.0	66	10	1.0

[a]CHO, carbohydrates.
[b]Sweet powders made up with whole milk.

Nuts

In the popular sense the term 'nut' is applied to a seed or fruit with an edible kernel inside a brittle or hard shell; the botanical definition is somewhat more complicated.

The species to be discussed in the present account are: hazel or cob (*Corylus avellana*), filbert (*Corylus maxima*), sweet or Spanish chestnut (*Castanea sativa*), almond (*Prunus dulcis* syn. *P. amygdalus*, *Amygdalus communis*), common or Persian walnut (*Juglans regia*), black walnut (*Juglans nigra*), white walnut or butternut (*Juglans cinerea*), pistachio (*Pistacia vera*), pecan (*Carya pecan* syn. *C. illinoensis*), Brazil nut (*Bertholletia excelsa*), cashew nut (*Anacardium occidentale*), pine kernels (*Pinus* species.), Queensland or macadamia nut (*Macadamia integrifolia*, smooth shelled; *M. tetraphylla*, rough shelled), peanut or monkey nut or groundnut (*Arachis hypogaea*), and coconut (*Cocos nucifera*).

ORIGIN AND CULTIVATION

Nuts have long been an item in the human diet – remains have been found in archaeological sites dating back to before 10 000 BC. They were an important food item for the hunter-gatherers and were brought into cultivation at a very early date; it has been suggested that nut harvesting might have taken place before cultivation of cereals in agriculture. Most nut species are now cultivated, although Brazil nuts are harvested entirely in the wild. Collection of nuts from some other species in the wild (e.g. hazel) still takes place but this is usually as an addition to the normal diet.

Nut species are cultivated in temperate climates (e.g. hazel, filbert, sweet chestnut, almond, walnut species, pistachio, pecan) and in warmer climates (e.g. peanut, coconut).

PLANT DESCRIPTION

A large number of the nut species are trees, but peanut is an annual growing to a height of 15–60 cm (24 in).

CULINARY AND NUTRITIONAL VALUE

Nut kernels are consumed raw, roasted, or salted, or in a great variety of products, e.g. nut butters, confectionery, curries, soups, stews, snack foods, sweetmeats, flour, bread, porridge, poultry stuffing, fritters, animal feed, cake, ice-cream, sauces, puddings, and meat and fish dishes. Immature (green) kernels of some species (walnut, almond) may be eaten as such or pickled.

Some nut products have achieved a considerable reputation, e.g. 'groundnut (peanut) chop or stew' in West Africa, marrons glacé (sweet chestnut) in France, and pesto sauce (pine).

As with all food analyses of plant products, the results will vary according to the environment, the variety (cultivar), the method of analysis, and some other factors.

By and large, the major nutrients in nut kernels are protein and fat (oil). The exception is chestnut, where starch in the dried kernel could be as much as 60%, and the amounts of protein and fat are low. Protein quantities vary according to species, with as much as 30% in peanuts, but the average seems to be about 15%. High-protein peanut flour has been used to supplement milk beverages in India and to raise protein levels in bread and biscuits.

With the exception of coconut, which contains saturated fat, nut species contain unsaturated fat (polyunsaturated and monounsaturated). The amounts are high, ranging from about 50% (e.g. peanut, pistachio) to about 70% (e.g. Brazil nut, pecan, pine, macadamia, walnut).

Nuts are good sources of minerals – calcium, iron, magnesium, phosphorus, potassium, sodium, zinc, copper, manganese, and selenium. Naturally, a food analysis of salted nuts will give a high reading for sodium. Vitamins present are B_1, B_2, B_6, niacin, pantothenic acid, folate, and E. Vitamin C, not normally present in nuts, is found in green (immature) walnuts (1300–3000 mg per 100 g).

In reasonably recent times, interest has been shown in other substances present in nuts – flavonoids (quercetin and kaempferol) in almonds; resveratrol (a phytoalexin) in peanuts; sterols in pecans.

Nuts are a good source of dietary fibre (6–12 g per 100 g) and can be important commercial oilseeds (peanut, almond, coconut). The nutritional value of hazel and filbert is essentially the same, as is the nutritional value of the various walnut species.

CLAIMS AND FOLKLORE

Nuts have been used in medicine; e.g. tea made from peanuts has been used in Mexico and Peru to stimulate milk production in nursing mothers, and in Brazil as a nerve tonic; in Vietnam almonds are employed to cure dysentery.

However, as a health food, nuts provide a range of important nutrients such as protein, fat, minerals, vitamins, and dietary fibre. High intakes of saturated fat have been associated with heart disease and certain cancers (see p. xvii); therefore, nut unsaturated fat is to be considered 'healthy'. The role of antioxidants in dealing with free radicals and heart disease has already been described (see p. xvii). Nuts include antioxidants such as vitamin E, flavonoids, and certain trace elements such as selenium; Brazil nut is a rich source of this element (153 µg per 100 g). In animal and human experiments, plant sterols (which reportedly occur

Nuts

in some nut species) have been shown to reduce total cholesterol and its low-density lipoprotein fraction. Resveratrol, found in peanut skins and kernels, is also found in grape skins and red wine. The 'French paradox' postulates that those who consume red wine regularly, even with a high fat diet, have less incidence of coronary heart disease than inhabitants of England and Wales. Resveratrol, a phytoalexin, could contribute to this situation, but other substances, e.g. flavonoids, might be responsible.

EVIDENCE

It has previously been pointed out (see p. xvii) that unsaturated fat and antioxidants are good for general health. In addition, the presence of other substances, e.g. flavonoids, render nuts a good health food. Also, as in all other plant materials, nuts are cholesterol free. However, as has been stated, nuts are rich in fats, and about 30 g (1 oz) of kernels provide 200 kcal – a sizeable fraction of a normal day's requirement. Therefore, there must be some control of the amount of nuts in a diet. There are those who claim that nuts constitute a 'satiety' factor – they limit the amount of food consumed; however, there is sometimes a feeling that nuts are 'moreish'.

A number of human epidemiological studies in the USA claim that frequent nut eaters have a lower risk of heart disease than non-consumers. Also, other studies claim that nuts in the diet reduce total blood cholesterol and the low-density lipoprotein fraction while not affecting the high-density lipoprotein fraction.

One of the difficulties associated with the consumption of nuts is that they may cause allergies – peanut is notorious in this respect. In extreme cases peanuts can bring about anaphylaxis, which can be fatal or near fatal. Those who are aware that they are allergic to peanuts obviously must avoid them, but it can be difficult because a wide range of products do contain peanuts or peanut oil, e.g. biscuits, cakes, ice-cream desserts, cereal bars, curries, and many others. Peanut oil is used in cosmetics. Discussion has taken place about the relative safety of unrefined and refined peanut oil. It is the peanut protein that is responsible for the allergy and therefore a refined oil might well be safe, but those who are allergic should consider the wisdom of ingesting the oil. Considerable efforts are now made in food outlets and by manufacturers to warn of the danger of nuts.

Under certain conditions, peanuts may become infected with the moulds (fungi) *Aspergillus flavus* and *A. parasiticus*. These moulds can produce chemicals (mycotoxins) known as 'aflatoxins', which are carcinogenic. The situation is being carefully monitored in a number of countries (e.g. UK, USA, and others) because infected nuts must not enter the food chain. In the UK, the limit for aflatoxin is 4 µg per kg in finished peanut products and 10 µg per kg in products intended for further processing before sale (1 µg = 0.001 mg).

Temperate and tropical nuts are illustrated in *The new Oxford book of food plants* (Vaughan and Geissler; see recommended reading list).

Orris *Iris germanica var. florentina;* blue flag *Iris versicolor*

Family Iridaceae

ORIGIN AND CULTIVATION

Orris is a native of southern Italy but naturalized in central Europe, Iran, and northern India. It is cultivated commercially, particularly in Italy. Several other species (e.g. *Iris pallida*) are grown as sources of orris.

Orris is best known as a scent and fixative source, being used in perfumery, pot pourris, shampoos, and dusting powders. The plant part used is the rhizome or rootstock, although the product is normally referred to as orris root. The violet scent, which intensifies as the rhizome ages, is related to an essential oil consisting partly of irone. It has been claimed that the rhizome was used in ancient Egypt, Greece, and Rome, although it has been suggested that the plant was first cultivated in medieval Florence.

I. versicolor is a native of North America.

PLANT DESCRIPTION

Orris is a perennial with a rhizome up to 5 cm (2 in) thick. The plant grows to a height of 60–120 cm (4 ft), and has sword-shaped leaves and white, violet-tinged flowers.

Blue flag is a similar plant but has larger leaves and purple, yellow-veined flowers.

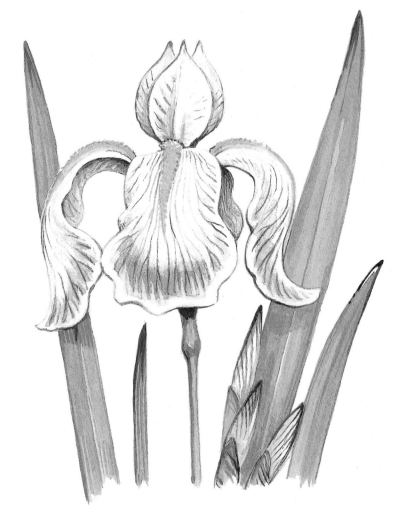

CULINARY AND NUTRITIONAL VALUE
None.

CLAIMS AND FOLKLORE

Orris rhizome has had a number of herbal uses, e.g. as a diuretic, expectorant, purgative, and antidiarrhoeal.

Blue flag rhizome, used by native North Americans, has had a number of applications: it has been used externally to treat skin diseases, rheumatism, and infected wounds, and

internally, psoriasis, acne, herpes, migraine, and some other conditions.

EVIDENCE

Little is known about the properties of these iris species, although rhizome extracts can cause nausea and vomiting. The plants seem little used at present for medicinal purposes and are probably best avoided, including during pregnancy. No support is given to the herb in Germany.

Parsley piert *Aphanes arvensis*

Family Rosaceae

ORIGIN AND CULTIVATION
The plant grows in waste places and on wall tops, being widely distributed in Europe, Ethiopia, central Asia, Australia, and North America.

PLANT DESCRIPTION
Parsley piert is a small annual rarely more than 8 cm (3 in) high. It is much branched, green, and hairy. Flowers are very small and may be produced when the plant is only about 2 cm ($\frac{4}{5}$ in) in height.

The whole plant is used to prepare herbal medicine. It should not be confused with parsley (*Petroselinum crispum*), which is a very important food herb.

CULINARY AND NUTRITIONAL VALUE
In the Scottish Hebrides, it was once eaten as a salad vegetable, or pickled for winter use.

CLAIMS AND FOLKLORE
Parsley piert is astringent, demulcent, and can act as a diuretic. Plant extracts have been used to treat urinary infections, bladder and kidney stones, and urinary gravel.

EVIDENCE
No direct evidence is available concerning its chemical constituents, but because of its astringent nature it probably contains tannins (tannins are recorded for the related lady's mantle, *Alchemilla vulgaris*).

No experiments are recorded. Because of the lack of data concerning toxicity, care should be taken with parsley piert, particularly during pregnancy and lactation.

Peppermint *Mentha × piperita*

Family Labiatae/Lamiaceae

ORIGIN AND CULTIVATION

Peppermint is a hybrid of *Mentha aquatica* (water mint) and *M. spicata* (spearmint). It is a native of Europe and Asia and naturalized in North America. The plant grows in hedgerows, on waste ground, and on banks of streams. It is cultivated in a number of European countries, North Africa, and the USA.

PLANT DESCRIPTION

The plant has lanceolate, ovate, short-stalked leaves up to 8 cm (3 in) long, and terminal, oblong spikes of flowers, their stamens more or less concealed within the reddish lilac corolla. It grows to a height of 30–90 cm (3 ft).

Its importance lies in the production of peppermint oil by distillation. The whole plant and its oil are employed.

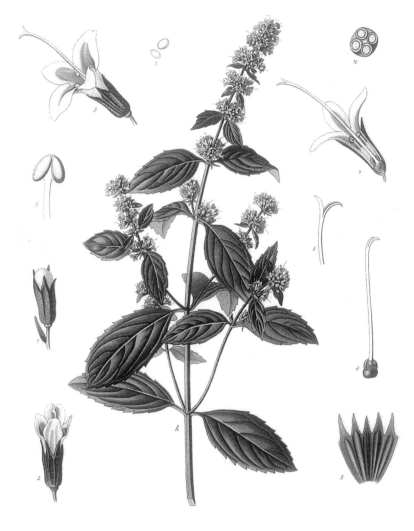

CULINARY AND NUTRITIONAL USES

Peppermint produces 0.1–1% of an essential oil, of which menthol is a major constituent, although there are many others. It is used in confectionery, ice-cream, chewing gum, liqueurs (e.g. crème de menthe), perfumery, and cigarettes.

CLAIMS AND FOLKLORE

Peppermint is claimed to be of value for problems of the digestive system such as wind, indigestion, gastroenteritis, and irritable bowel syndrome. Peppermint is used as an inhalant and chest rub for respiratory infections. It may be applied to the skin to relieve pain, headaches, and migraine.

EVIDENCE

Some experiments indicate that the oil is antimicrobial (*in vitro*), antiviral, antispasmodic (therefore of value in digestive problems), and anti-inflammatory. There is support for the herb and its oil in Germany.

Menthol in the oil may cause allergic reactions. Peppermint should not be given to young children. Indeed, the oil should not be taken internally except under close supervision.

Pilewort, lesser celandine *Ranunculus ficaria syn. Ficaria verna*

Family Ranunculaceae

ORIGIN AND CULTIVATION
Pilewort is a very common weed, found in fields, pastures, and waste places, and is distributed throughout Europe, western Asia, and North Africa.

PLANT DESCRIPTION
It has smooth and shining heart-shaped leaves. The roots are tuberous and the flowers yellow. Pilewort is 5–15 cm (6 in) high.

The complete plant is used to prepare herbal medicine.

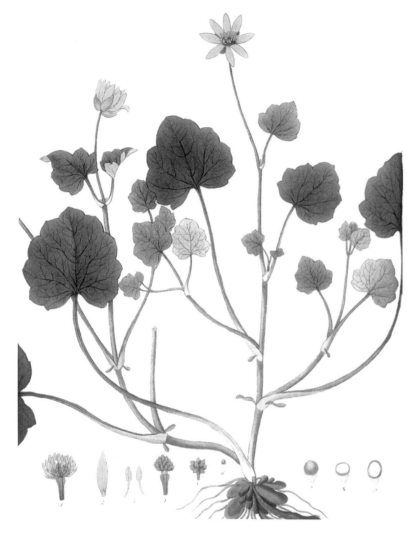

CULINARY AND NUTRITIONAL VALUE
None.

CLAIMS AND FOLKLORE
According to the medieval Doctrine of Signatures the tuberous roots of the plant resembled haemorrhoids (piles) and, therefore, extracts of the plant should have a healing effect.

In fact, being it is astringent and demulcent, this has been its main use and it is applied externally as an ointment.

EVIDENCE
Pilewort contains saponins and tannins. Animal studies have supported the value of the saponins for treating piles. The herbal extract should not be taken internally.

Pineapple *Ananas comosus*

Family Bromeliaceae

ORIGIN AND CULTIVATION
Pineapple was domesticated in tropical
South America in pre-Columbian times; it
is now widely grown in tropical and
subtropical countries, the major producing
areas being the USA, Mexico, Formosa,
Thailand, the Philippines, Malaysia, Ivory
Coast, South Africa, and Australia.

PLANT DESCRIPTION
It is a perennial or biennial, up to 1.5 m
(5 ft) in height, with tough spiny leaves.
The inflorescence of up to 200 reddish
purple flowers gives rise to the well known
fruit – usually about 20 cm (8 in) long and
14 cm (6 in) in diameter.

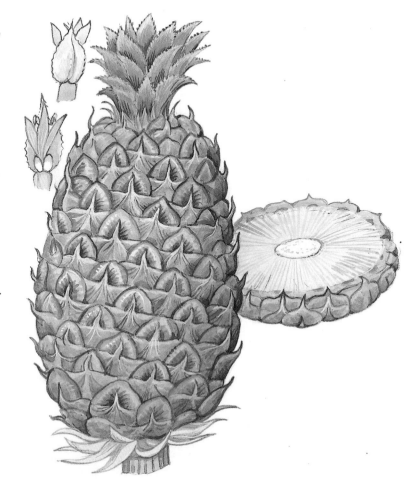

CULINARY AND NUTRITIONAL VALUE
Pineapples are a common fruit, being available fresh,
canned, and in the form of juice. The fresh fruit contains
about 10% total sugars – half of this is sucrose, the rest glucose and fructose. Dried pineapple has almost 70% sugars.
The vitamin C content of fresh fruit is 12 mg per 100 g, but
there is only a trace in the dried fruit.

Both the fruit and the stem contain the protein-digest-
ing enzyme bromelain. This has been used to prevent a
proteinaceous haze in chill-proof beer when refrigerated,
and to tenderize meat and modify dough.

CLAIMS AND FOLKLORE
The fruit has had a long history in traditional tropical
medicine, being used to improve digestion, increase
appetite, relieve dyspepsia (unripe fruit), and to act as a
diuretic (ripe fruit).

Bromelain has been included in preparations that are
claimed to be therapeutic as regards inflammation,
wounds, and infections, and in some diets that are alleged
to enhance fat excretion.

EVIDENCE
There does not seem to be much experimental support for the
above claims, but some animal experiments provide a little
support for the wound-healing claim. Obviously more work is
required. There is some approval for the fruit in Germany.

Side-effects, after pineapple ingestion, have included
uterine contractions, nausea, vomiting, diarrhoea, and
skin rash.

Plantain, psyllium, ispaghula, fleawort

various Plantago species

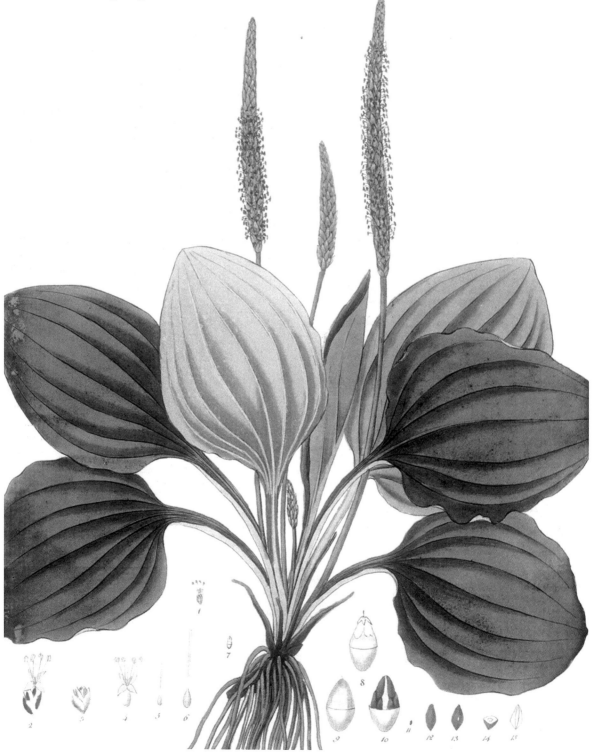

Plantain, psyllium, ispaghula, fleawort

Family Plantaginaceae

ORIGIN AND CULTIVATION

There are about 250 *Plantago* species. A number of these have been used medicinally, including *P. asiatica, P. ovata, P. psyllium, P. indica, P. arenaria, P. major,* and *P. lanceolata,* although not all these Latin names are accepted by botanists. According to species, they are found in Europe, North Africa, temperate Asia, and North America; there is cultivation of at least some species. *P. lanceolata* and *P. major* have been widely spread by human colonization, particularly by Europeans – in New Zealand plantain has been referred to by the Maoris as Englishman's foot.

PLANT DESCRIPTION

The plantain species are annuals, biennials, or perennials. Their general structure consists of a basal rosette of leaves up to 15 cm (6 in) in length, producing a single stem or spike bearing small greenish flowers, which, after fertilization, give rise to capsules containing the seeds of various colours. *P. indica* is an exception in that the flowering stem is branched.

Plantago should not be confused with the tropical genus *Musa,* which produces cooking bananas (plantains).

The parts utilized in herbal medicine are the leaves and seeds.

CULINARY AND NUTRITIONAL VALUE

The seed mucilage has been used as a thickener or stabilizer in certain frozen dairy desserts.

CLAIMS AND FOLKLORE

Plantain was first recorded in Chinese medicine during the Han dynasty (206 BC to AD 23).

Seed

Seeds contain up to 30% mucilage. Because of this, the seeds, their husks, or the refined mucilage are used in commercial bulk laxatives. It has also been claimed that such preparations might reduce total blood cholesterol, improve the high-density lipoprotein to low-density lipoprotein ratio, provide increased fibre in weight loss products, and improve irritable bowel syndrome. In addition, it has an antidiarrhoeal action, and is said to be valuable in the treatment of haemorrhoids in that it softens the stool and reduces irritation of the distended vein.

Pulverized seeds have been mixed with oil and applied to inflamed areas in the skin (including the eye), and mixed with honey for sore throats.

Leaves (or whole plant)

In herbal practice, leaves have been used externally to treat bruises, wounds (to stop bleeding), haemorrhoids, and ulcers. Internally, plantain has been involved in the treatment of acute infections of the lungs and urinary tract, hepatitis, diarrhoea, and boils.

EVIDENCE

The chemical constituents have been well documented, and there have been a number of animal and human studies. Its reputed effect in slowing down bleeding from wounds has been attributed to the tannins present. Aucubin (an iridoid glycoside) has been claimed as the active principle involved in liver protection. The results of scientific and clinical investigations into the use of plantain in dealing with bronchitis have been satisfactory enough to warrant further research.

Excessive use of plantain should be avoided during pregnancy.

Prickly ash (northern) *Zanthoxylum americanum;*
prickly ash (southern) *Zanthoxylum clava-herculis*

Family Rutaceae

ORIGIN AND CULTIVATION

Northern prickly ash is found in moist woodlands in southern Canada, and northern, central, and western parts of the USA; southern prickly ash grows in central and southern USA.

Other species utilized are *Zanthoxylum piperitum* (China), *Z. capense* (South Africa), and *Z. zanthoxyloides* (West Africa).

PLANT DESCRIPTION

Z. americanum, sometimes known as the toothache tree, is a deciduous shrub growing to a height of 4–8 m (26 ft). Its branches are spiny with pinnately divided leaves. The small yellow–green flowers give rise to tiny black fruits.

The parts used in herbal medicine are the bark and fruits.

CULINARY AND NUTRITIONAL VALUE

Extracts may have been used as food flavours.

CLAIMS AND FOLKLORE

Although the chemical compositions for *Z. americanum* and *Z. clava-herculis* are slightly different their herbal uses are the same, as treatments for toothache, rheumatism, fever, arthritis, and poor digestion.

EVIDENCE

Both species contain alkaloids (isoquinoline), resins, tannins, and essential oil, but there are differences; e.g. coumarins are recorded for *Z. americanum*.

There has been limited experimental work concerning the efficacy of prickly ash so excessive use should be avoided. It would probably be wise not to use the herbal during pregnancy and lactation.

Probiotics

Products such as 'live' or 'bio' or 'probiotic' drinks or yoghurts are now available in increasing variety. Probiotic bacteria may also be available in capsules or as powder.

The concept of probiotics is not a new one. Early in the twentieth century the Nobel Prize winner Elie Metchnikoff observed the longevity of Bulgarian peasants and suggested that this was due to their high intake of 'soured milks' – the predecessors of the probiotic drinks and yoghurts being sold now. The ideas he expressed went out of fashion but are now being explored by the scientific community.

In the human gastrointestinal tract, mainly in the colon, there are a huge number of bacteria, without which the functions of the digestive tract would be virtually impossible. These bacteria colonize the gut soon after birth and live on the undigested remains of foods passing through the gastrointestinal tract. Although we are still learning about the functions of these bacteria, it is possible that they may play an important part in maintaining human health.

Some of the bacterial species may be thought of as harmful – e.g. they may cause gastroenteritis and may possibly be involved in other chronic disorders such as inflammatory bowel disease. Others, mainly *Bifidobacter* and *Lactobacillus* species, are thought to exert protective effects in the gut. There is currently much interest in the possibility of increasing the proportion of the 'beneficial' bacteria at the expense of those that may be harmful. It is thought that this may be achieved either by (a) adding probiotic bacteria to foods, or (b) stimulating their growth, by providing specific undigested food components, called prebiotics.

The most commonly used definition of probiotics is that they are 'live microbial food ingredients that are beneficial to health', a phrase which reflects the fact that these materials are increasingly being added to milk and dairy products to produce 'functional foods'.

In order to be classified as a probiotic for use in human food, a bacterial species must:

- be of human origin;
- be non-pathogenic;
- tolerate acid and bile;
- remain viable over the whole shelf-life of the product;
- show evidence of beneficial effects in human studies.

Probiotic bacteria must be able to resist digestion or destruction by stomach acid and bile in order to reach the large intestine, and must, to be effective, either stick to the lining of the colon or colonize it. This requires very large numbers of bacteria (measured in 'colony forming units' and abbreviated to cfu) to be present in the food at the point when it is eaten. Studies have shown that many so-called probiotic or 'bio' yoghurts do not satisfy this requirement. In the UK at present yoghurts labelled 'live' or 'bio' may contain live bacterial cultures but not necessarily probiotic bacteria, and if such cultures are added they may not be present in appropriate quantities.

The sour milk or yoghurt drinks seem to result in better delivery of appropriate numbers of probiotic bacteria than bio-yoghurts, but even these have to be taken daily in order to make sure that the bacteria are constantly present in the gut. In the US the National Yoghurt Association (NYA) is involved in a scheme that certifies that yoghurts meet the criteria for live and active cultures.

The most common bacteria used in probiotic products are shown in Table 25. They are mostly characterized as lactic-acid producing bacteria, although some *Bacillus* species may be probiotic, as may some fungi (*Saccharomyces* species and *Aspergillus* species).

Table 25 Bacteria that are alleged to have probiotic activity

Lactobacilli	Bifidobacteria	Others
L. acidophilus[a]	B. animalis	Bacillus cereus
L. casei	B. breve	Escheichia coli
L. johnsonii	B. infantis	Streptococcus boulardii
L. reuteri	B. longum	Clostridium butyricum
L. rhamnosus	B. adolescentis	Enterococcus faecium
L. salvarius	B. lactis	
L. plantarum	B. bifidum	
L. crispatus		

[a] L., Lactobacillus, B., Bifidobacter.

Sometimes probiotic bacteria are sold in capsules or as part of vitamin supplements. However, it is thought that survival in the gut is better if they are taken as yoghurt or sour milk drinks.

PROPOSED BENEFICIAL EFFECTS OF CONSUMING PROBIOTICS

There are a great many claims made for benefits, some of which have more substantiation than others. Manufacturers of 'probiotic' products claim that they help to 'balance' the intestinal bacteria, i.e. ensure that there are more 'good' bacteria than 'bad' and hence help protect the

Probiotics

gut. An expert review of the scientific literature recently concluded that more evidence is required for most claims, but that some probiotics may help prevent diarrhoea due to bacterial or virus infection, and may shorten the length of the diarrhoeal phase in certain gastrointestinal infections in children. Some studies have shown that probiotics improve digestion of lactose in people who are intolerant to this. Some studies have shown a reduction in blood cholesterol levels while consuming probiotics, but others using the same products have not. Studies suggesting that consumption strengthens the immune system are accumulating, but it is difficult to assess what benefits this might have as a whole range of different measures of immune stimulation are being used. There is as yet insufficient evidence supporting the claims that probiotic consumption prevents cancer.

PREBIOTICS

These have been defined as 'non-digestible food ingredients that beneficially affect the host by selectively stimulating the growth and/or activity of one or a limited number of bacteria in the colon that can improve the host health'. They therefore encourage the growth of lactic-acid producing organisms such as lactobacilli and bifidobacteria that are already present in the gut. The majority of prebiotics are oligosaccharides (short-chain carbohydrates) of the monosaccharides fructose or galactose. Lactulose, an indigestible disaccharide sometimes prescribed as a laxative, may also act as a prebiotic. Other potential prebiotics include oligosaccharides from soya beans and a variety of man-made oligosaccharides. Inulin, found in Jerusalem artichokes, is a prebiotic that has been used to study the effects of these materials, and you will also sometimes see or hear the term 'FOS' (fructo-oligosaccharides). Most of the substances now presented as prebiotics certainly provide a substrate for gut bacteria. The presence of these and similar materials has often been given as the explanation for the flatulence experienced after consumption of such foods as onions, beans, or Jerusalem artichokes; this occurs when the bacteria ferment the carbohydrate that our own enzymes cannot break down.

The most common use for prebiotics, especially inulin, at the moment is as a dietary fibre, bulking agent, and fat replacer in foods, and in future the food uses are likely to increase. There have been few studies of the potential benefits, and although a mixture of oligosaccharides, including inulin, has been shown in one study to lower plasma cholesterol, further research will be necessary to investigate other beneficial effects.

In some countries 'synbiotics' (a mixture of prebiotic material and probiotic bacterial culture) are being added to foods. The assumption here is that the prebiotic will encourage the growth of the accompanying bacteria in the gut. So you might have prebiotic FOS in a food together with a *Bifidobacter* species. However, research is still needed to find appropriate mixtures, as different bacteria may need different prebiotics to be effective.

Pulsatilla, pasque flower
Pulsatilla vulgaris syn. Anemone pulsatilla

Family Ranunculaceae

ORIGIN AND CULTIVATION

Pulsatilla is found growing in pastures throughout temperate Eurasia and North Africa, but is now rare in the wild because of overharvesting and loss of habitat. A number of *Pulsatilla* species are used in herbal medicine throughout the world.

PLANT DESCRIPTION

It is a perennial with a thick rootstock. The leaves are finely divided and, like the stems and flowers, covered with soft hairs. Its bell-shaped flower is dark purple, about 3 cm (1 in) in length, and gives rise to feathery fruits. It grows to a height of 10–25 cm (10 in).

The aerial parts are used in herbal medicine.

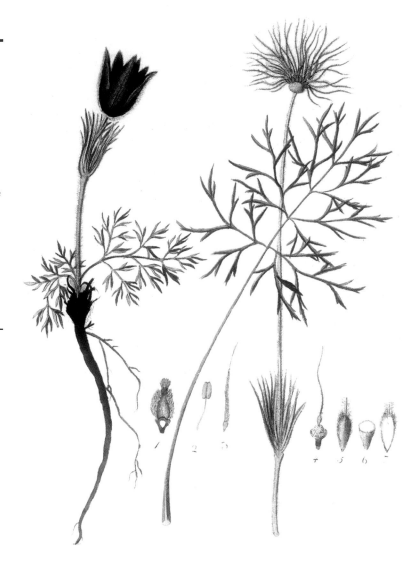

CULINARY AND NUTRITIONAL VALUE

None.

CLAIMS AND FOLKLORE

Pulsatilla extracts have been used particularly for problems of the female and male reproductive systems, e.g. premenstrual syndrome, period pains (especially when accompanied by nervous exhaustion), and epididymitis. The drug has also been employed as a sedative and for treating coughs. It is frequently found in homeopathic remedies.

EVIDENCE

Among the chemical compounds present in the plant are flavonoids, saponins, and essential oils. The drug should be treated with caution because excess can lead to diarrhoea, vomiting, and convulsions; it should only be used under the direction of a qualified herbalist. Fresh plant material must be avoided because it contains the poisonous protoanemonin, which in dried material degrades to the non-toxic anemonin.

Pulsatilla should not be taken during pregnancy and lactation. It is not approved in Germany.

Pulses, peas, beans, and lentils *legumes*

The Leguminosae (Fabaceae) is one of the largest families of flowering plants (over 15 000 species), ranging from tiny wild plants to large trees. Members of the family can easily be recognized by (a) the flower with its petals comprising a large upper standard, two lateral wings, and a boat-shaped keel, and (b) the fruit, known as the legume or pod, containing the seeds or beans.

As regards a source of food (human and animal) on a world basis it is second only to the grasses (cereals). Food types from the family include dry seeds (pulses), green pods, immature green seeds, sprouts (germinated seeds), spices, and oilseeds.

Pulses are widely sold in health shops, stores, and supermarkets. Soya (*Glycine max*) is described on p. 146, and groundnut (*Arachis hypogaea*) on p. 115.

ORIGIN AND CULTIVATION

Crops cultivated for pulses are found in temperate and tropical areas. They are of ancient origin and, indeed, are some of the oldest crops known to the human race. It is of interest that there is parallel domestication between legumes and cereals: (a) wheat, barley, pea, lentil, broad bean, and chick-pea in west Asia and Europe; (b) maize and common bean in America; (c) pearl millet, sorghum, and cowpea in Africa; and (d) rice and soya bean in China.

Some species can be grown in areas of low rainfall and poor soil. Most pulses are now cultivated in many countries – they are no longer restricted to their centres of origin. Some well known pulses are as follows:

- Mat- or moth-bean of India (*Vigna aconitifolia* syn. *Phaseolus aconitifolius*). Cultivated in India, Pakistan, Burma, China, USA, and other countries. Seeds are rectangular to cylindrical (3–5×1.5–2.5 mm), light brown, whitish green, or yellow–brown.

- Adzuki bean (*Vigna angularis* syn. *Phaseolus angularis*). Cultivated in Japan, Korea, Manchuria, India, and other countries. The pulse is included in soups, cakes, and confectionery, and is germinated to give sprouts. Seeds (5–7.5 ×4.55 mm) are red creamish, black, or mottled.

- Tepary bean (*Phaseolus acutifolius*). Cultivated in Mexico, USA, Africa, Asia, and Australia. The pulse is included in soup. Seeds (8×6 mm) are white, yellow, brown, or deep violet.

- Rice-bean (*Vigna umbellata* syn. *Phaseolus calcaratus*). Cultivated in China, Korea, Japan, and India. The pulse is eaten with rice or instead of rice. Seeds (5–10×2–5 mm) are oblong to elongate and red, green, yellow, brown, or black.

- Runner bean (*Phaseolus coccineus* syn. *P. multiflorus*). Domesticated in Mexico and introduced into Europe in the sixteenth century. In its area of origin, it is cultivated for tender pods, green and dry seeds, and starchy roots. The crop is now grown for pods and pulses in highland areas of Africa and South America, and for pods in temperate lands. Seeds (variable in size) are ovoid and pink to purple, mottled, or sometimes black, white, cream, or brown.

- Common bean (*Phaseolus vulgaris*). This is the best known and most widely cultivated bean in the world. Archaeological remains, dated about 5000 BC, have been found in Mexico. It was introduced into Europe by the Spaniards and Portuguese in the sixteenth century – and to Africa and other parts of the Old World. The plant is the main pulse crop in tropical America and many parts of tropical Africa. In temperate areas it is grown mainly for the young pods.

  In addition to common, this bean has a host of other names: French, kidney, haricot, snap, frijoles, berlotto, cannellino, pinto, pea-bean, navy, marrow, black bean, flageolet. Seeds vary in shape (kidney to globose), size (7–18 mm in length) and colour (black, white, red, buff, brown, or combinations of these colours).

  These beans have been included in some famous food products and dishes, e.g. canned baked beans in tomato sauce; French cassoulet (beans with meat pieces); red kidney beans in chilli con carne; cannellino beans with tuna fish in tonno e fagioli (Italy).

- Butter bean, Lima bean, Madagascar bean (*Phaseolus lunatus*). Found in many tropical, subtropical, and warm temperate areas of America, Africa, and Asia. The seeds are variable in size (1–3 cm in length) and colour (white, cream, red, purple, brown, black, mottled). Its dry seeds are utilized as pulses, and the green immature beans are eaten. They may be canned or frozen. The pulse provides a protein-rich flour used in bread and noodles in the Philippines and bean paste in Japan. The seeds may be germinated to give 'sprouts'.

- Chick-pea (*Cicer arietinum*). Produced in considerable amounts in India, the Middle East, and the Mediterranean region. The beaked seeds are white, yellow, red, brown, or nearly black. Chick-pea can be used for 'dhal' (associated with curry), and the seed flour is found in many forms of Indian confectionery. In the Mediterranean region the cooked pulses plus sesame oil and other flavourings are included in a well known side-dish 'hummus' – and also 'falafel'.

- Black gram, Urd (*Vigna mungo* syn. *Phaseolus mungo*). Cultivated in India, South-east Asia, East Africa, West Indies, and USA. The seeds are black or olive green. The seeds are treated as pulses, boiled or eaten whole, and also included in 'dhal'. Seed flour is included in porridge, bread, and biscuits. In Japan the seed is germinated to give 'sprouts'. The plant is drought resistant.

Pulses, peas, beans, and lentils

- Mung bean, golden gram, green gram (*Vigna radiata* syn. *Phaseolus aureus*). Cultivated in India and elsewhere. The seeds are usually green but sometimes yellow or black. The dried beans are cooked, then eaten whole or used, often split, in 'dhal'. They can be milled to give a flour, found in soups, porridge, snacks, bread, noodles, and even ice-cream. The seed starch is used to make starch noodles and its protein used to fortify cereal flours. Mung bean seed is said to cause less flatulence than other legumes. All pulses can be germinated to give sprouts, which may be eaten raw or cooked and are popular in salads and oriental cooking, but mung bean is the most widely used in North America, Asia, and Europe.

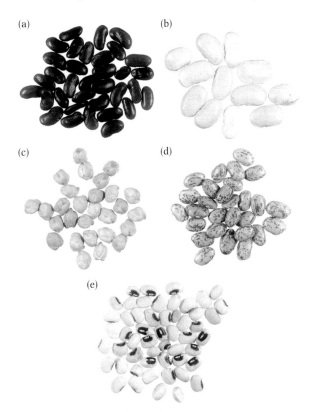

(a) Red kidney beans. (b) Butter beans. (c) Chick-peas. (d) Pinto beans. (e) Black-eyed beans.

- Faba, broad bean (*Vicia faba*). Cultivated in many countries with a temperate climate. The seeds are variable in shape and colour (white, green, buff, brown, purple, black) and 6–30 mm in length. Immature green seeds are cooked as a vegetable, or canned or frozen. Dry mature seeds (pulses) constitute human food or animal feed. In Egypt, the seeds are a popular food known as 'foul'.

- Pea (*Pisum sativum*). Grown in temperate regions, the subtropics (cool season), and tropics (high altitude). The seeds are very variable as regards surface features (round or wrinkled) and colour (green, brownish, white, blue). Dry seeds were utilized as food in Europe from early days, but green peas were not used until the sixteenth century. In the UK well known dry peas are green 'marrowfats' and 'split yellow' (which has a white seed coat). Petit pois are small and very acceptable green peas. Dry seeds (pulses) (whole, split, or ground into flour) are cooked and used in soups, pease pudding, and convenience foods, or rehydrated and canned ('processed peas'). Seed coats (hulls) are added as fibre to bread and health foods, and pea protein is added to increase both amount and quality of protein in such foods. Green or immature seeds are cooked as a vegetable and are often canned or frozen. The seeds are particularly free of toxic constituents.

- Lentil (*Lens culinaris* syn. *L. esculenta*). The Indian subcontinent is the largest producer but it is also grown in most subtropical and warm temperate countries. On sale as pulses, the seeds are biconvex or lens-shaped (3–9 mm in length) and green, yellow, orange, red, or brown in colour. The pulses, entire or split, are used in soups and 'dhal'; they can be fried, seasoned, and consumed as snack food. Flour made from pulses can be mixed with cereals in cakes, and invalid and infant food. Lentil pulses have few antinutritional factors.

- Cowpea, black-eyed bean (*Vigna unguiculata*). Cultivated in West Africa, Brazil, Texas, Georgia, and California. The seed is variable in shape (square to oblong) and size (5–10×4–8 mm). Colours also vary – buff, brown, red, black, or white (white seeds have pigment confined to a narrow eye, and hence are often described as black-eyed beans). Immature seeds can be canned or frozen. The pulse is included in soup and cakes (deep fried or steamed).

- Grass-pea or chickling vetch (*Lathyrus sativus*). Grown mainly in the Indian subcontinent and can tolerate dry places and poor soils. In India, it is the cheapest pulse available. The seeds are white, brown, or mottled, with flattened sides (diameter 4–7 mm). The pulse is boiled in water and eaten; it is also found in chapattis, paste balls, and curries. It is consumed by the very poor in times of famine. If the seeds are eaten over a prolonged period, they can cause 'lathyrism' – paralysis of the lower limbs (the main causative agent is a non-protein amino acid: beta-oxalyl-diamino-propionic acid).

Pulses, peas, beans, and lentils

NUTRITIONAL VALUE

Pulses are good sources of protein (often over 20% – peanuts and soya beans are especially rich sources). The proteins in legumes generally contain substantial amounts of essential amino acids, including lysine, but have low amounts of the sulphur-containing amino acids, methionine and cystine (non-essential). Cereals have low amounts of lysine but adequate amounts of the sulphur amino acids, and dishes such as 'rice and peas', 'baked beans on toast', or 'kitchadi', which combine cereals and legumes, supply high-quality protein.

Most pulses provide carbohydrate, which is mostly starch with a small amount of sugars and oligosaccharides. The carbohydrate content is 13–65% with, in most species, starch constituting 40–55% of digestible carbohydrates, soya beans and peanuts being notable exceptions.

Most species are low in fat (1.0–2.5%) with the exception of chick-peas, peanuts, and soya beans. The fat is unsaturated (mainly polyunsaturated).

Pulses contain a range of minerals, including calcium, iron, magnesium, zinc, potassium, and copper, but have a low sodium content. They are a useful source of dietary fibre and the types of polysaccharides present have potentially beneficial effects. Although the phytic acid associated with the dietary fibre is also high, it is thought that this does not significantly reduce mineral absorption from mixed diets containing the foods. The legumes supply a range of water-soluble vitamins, including folates (but not, unless sprouted, vitamin C).

POTENTIAL BENEFITS

Legumes are a useful source of protein, provide a range of other nutrients in vegetarian diets, and are a good source of dietary fibre in any diet. Experimental feeding studies have demonstrated that including reasonable amounts of some beans (e.g. haricot beans, chick-peas, soya) in the diet on a daily basis will lower blood cholesterol levels, and this has been largely put down to the effects of certain non-starch polysaccharides in the foods. However, consumption of soya protein isolates has also been shown to lower cholesterol levels. Legumes also have a low glycaemic index; i.e. blood sugar levels rise slowly after consumption of meals containing them. This may be of benefit in a variety of conditions – particularly diabetes mellitus.

Beansprouts (immature shoots of dried beans that have been sprouted by placing them in water in daylight) are rich in vitamin C.

POTENTIAL PROBLEMS

Legumes contain a range of 'antinutrients' and toxic substances in the seed: (a) lectins or haemagglutinins: found in many species and can be the cause of nausea, vomiting, diarrhoea, and abdominal pain in humans; (b) cyanogenic glycosides: have been associated with cyanide poisoning in lima beans; (c) stachyose and raffinose: carbohydrates (oligosaccharides) responsible for flatulence, which are fermented by bacteria in the large intestine; (d) lathyrogens in *Lathyrus sativus*: see above; (e) digestive enzyme inhibitors: soya and some other legumes contain proteins which can reduce protein digestion and utilization in the consumer; (f) favism: consumption of broad beans (*Vicia faba*) may result in haemolytic anaemia in susceptible people (a genetic defect in the red blood cells), who are usually of Mediterranean or Middle Eastern origin.

Because of the situation described, dry pulses should be well cooked to destroy the toxins before consumption. Pulses for sale to the public often carry warnings about proper processing.

Pumpkin seed *Cucurbita pepo*

Family Cucurbitaceae

ORIGIN AND CULTIVATION

Pumpkin is of New World origin, and was widely distributed over central and northern Mexico and the south-west USA. Archaeological remains, dated about 8750 BC, have been found in Mexico. It was an integral part of the corn (maize) – bean – squash complex, the main diet of several pre-Columbian civilizations. In the sixteenth century it was taken to Europe, and later to the Middle East, Africa, and the Far East.

PLANT DESCRIPTION

The plant has a creeping stem or it may be bushy. Its leaves and stems are bristly and the leaves have a heart-shaped base. The yellow flowers are unisexual.

Pumpkin fruits can be large (8–12 kg in weight) or small (2.5–3 kg). The cream, yellow, or orange fruit flesh is used in pies; the fruits are associated with Hallowe'en.

Its seeds are frequently sold in health food outlets. These are bottle shaped, markedly ridged, cream in colour, and up to 2.5 cm (1 in) in length. However, in the early 1970s, in the USA, varieties (cultivars) were developed with naked seeds, i.e. without seed coats, although the thin inner part of the seed coat does remain. These naked seeds, frequently found in health food stores, are not markedly ridged and are often green in colour, due presumably to chlorophyll in the remaining inner part of the seed coat.

CULINARY AND NUTRITIONAL VALUE

The seeds are eaten like nuts, raw or roasted, or fried in deep fat and salted to give 'pepitos'. In some parts of Central America the roasted kernels are combined with a sticky syrup to form 'pepitorio', a sweet confection. The kernels are included in bakery products (e.g. bread, pies), breakfast cereals, and salads.

Oil is present in the seed to the extent of 40–50%. It contains 80% unsaturated fatty acids, of which 60% is linoleic acid. The oil is sometimes extracted (it is important in Austria) and used in salad dressing, sauces, and even cakes. It should not be used in frying because of its low burning point.

The seed contains 30–40% protein, and a range of minerals such as calcium, phosphorus (quite a lot), iron, magnesium, zinc, and others. Vitamins present include E, K, B, and other water-soluble types. Some analyses report vitamin A – this presumably relates to the carotenes present. There is about 2% fibre and 15% carbohydrate, giving, with other seed constituents, about 550 kcal per 100 g.

CLAIMS AND FOLKLORE

From what has been stated above, pumpkin seed would appear to be non-toxic and a good source of a range of nutrients.

It has been used for centuries in Latin America, Africa, and India in traditional medicine to immobilize and expel intestinal worms and parasites. The active ingredient appears to be 'cucurbitin' (0.18–0.66% in the seed).

Pumpkin seed has also been suggested as a soothing treatment for prostate and bladder problems.

EVIDENCE

While pumpkin seeds might be effective in dealing with intestinal worms and parasites, it is now generally replaced by more modern treatments.

As regards its use for urinary problems, it would be very advisable to seek medical advice before employing pumpkin.

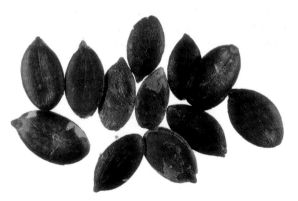

Quassia (Jamaican) *Picrasma excelsa syn. Picraenia excelsa;* quassia (Surinam) *Quassia amara*

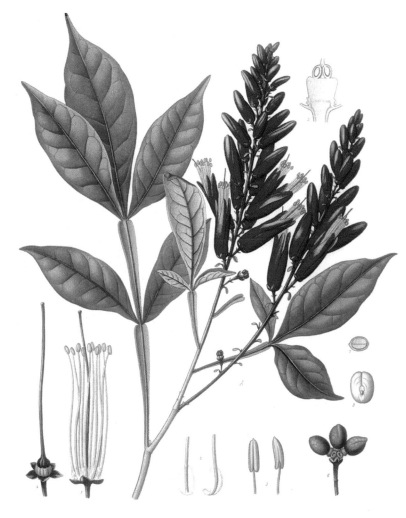

Family Simaroubaceae

ORIGIN AND CULTIVATION

These species are found in the West Indies, Central and South America, and other tropical countries. The wood was first imported into Europe in the latter part of the eighteenth century or the beginning of the nineteenth.

PLANT DESCRIPTION

- *Picrasma excelsa*: a tree growing to a height of 25 m (82 ft) and bearing pinnate leaves up to 30 cm (1 ft) in length. Its small green–white flowers give rise eventually to black berries.

- *Quassia amara*: a small tree up to 3 m (10 ft) in height.

CULINARY AND NUTRITIONAL VALUE

The bitter compounds (quassinoids) extracted from the wood (and bark) are terpenoids, and are 50 times more bitter than quinine. They are added to alcoholic and non-alcoholic beverages and some other food products, although there are limits to the quantities allowed.

CLAIMS AND FOLKLORE

Quassia has been used to treat lice, worms, malaria, and poor appetite, although an excess taken internally can cause nausea and vomiting.

EVIDENCE

One large human study supported the use of quassia to treat head lice, and it is probably useful as an appetite stimulant although there appears to be no evidence to support its antimalarial use. There should be caution concerning the quantities of quassia employed, and it should not be taken during pregnancy and lactation.

'Quorn' *The trade name for fungal protein or mycoprotein derived from* Fusarium graminearum

ORIGIN AND CULTIVATION

This product is derived from a tiny fungus (*Fusarium graminearum*) originally found in the early 1960s in fields near Marlow, Buckinghamshire, UK. The fungus is propagated by a continuous fermentation process; this gives a paste-like product known as mycoprotein, although, as described below, it contains nutrients in addition to protein (65–90% depending on product type). Other fungi of food importance include various mushrooms.

Table 26 Quorn: main nutrient content (per 100 g)

Water	75 g
Protein	11 g
Fat	3 g
Carbohydrate	3 g
Fibre	6 g
Ash (minerals)	2 g
Energy value	85 kcal

CULINARY AND NUTRITIONAL VALUE

Quorn products can be obtained as pieces, or ground (minced), sausages, burgers, steaks, etc. To manufacture these products, the mycoprotein is mixed after the fermentation process with small amounts of other ingredients, but is always meat free. It is therefore suitable for vegetarians.

Minerals present include appreciable amounts of calcium, magnesium, phosphorus, and potassium, and smaller amounts of copper, iron, manganese, sodium, and zinc.

The protein has a good amino acid profile, including all the essential ones. Unlike other 'protein' foods, Quorn contains dietary fibre (soluble and insoluble), which is present in a reasonable amount. Fat content is low, and there is a good ratio of polyunsaturated and monounsaturated fatty acids to saturated. Fungi are not always regarded as plants but there is no cholesterol in Quorn.

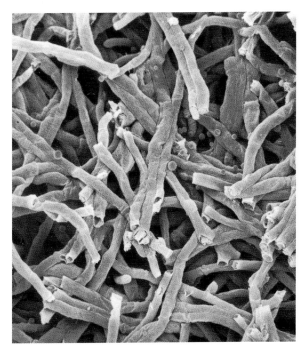

An electron microscope picture of Quorn, showing fungal threads (hyphae).

Quorn is therefore regarded as a 'healthy' food. Furthermore, its texture resembles that of meat, which is useful in the formulation of products such as 'steaks' or 'fillets'.

Some preliminary clinical studies have been carried out that indicate that Quorn might (a) reduce total and low-density lipoprotein blood cholesterol and occasionally raise high-density lipoprotein levels; (b) be of benefit in the dietary treatment of diabetes and have an effect on satiety; i.e. a lunch containing mycoprotein, compared with a control lunch, would reduce the amount of food consumed in the evening.

Raspberry *Rubus idaeus*

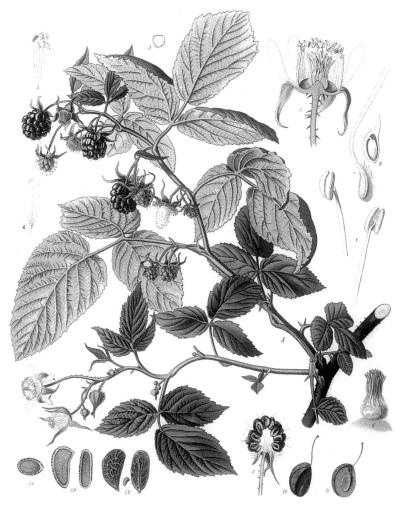

Family Rosaceae

ORIGIN AND CULTIVATION
Raspberry grows wild in Europe and western Asia, and was first introduced into cultivation almost 500 years ago in Europe. In North America, the wild raspberry is sometimes known as *Rubus strigosus* and was used by the early settlers; it was eventually domesticated.

PLANT DESCRIPTION
The stems, up to 1.5 m (5 ft) in height, are erect, with prickles; the leaves have 3–7 leaflets. Flowers are white, giving rise to downy red fruits.

The leaf is used in herbal medicine.

CULINARY AND NUTRITIONAL VALUE
Raspberry fruits are used for dessert, canning, freezing, purées, preserves, juice, jam (they are rich in pectin), jelly, bakery products, and a limited amount of wine.

The fruit contains 5–6% sugar, citric and some malic acid, and 13–38 mg vitamin C per 100 g.

CLAIMS AND FOLKLORE
The leaf contains, apart from other chemical constituents, tannins and flavonoids. Extracts, such as tea, have been used to treat diarrhoea, presumably because of its astringency. It has long been taken during the last 3 months of pregnancy, not in early pregnancy, to strengthen the uterus and ease childbirth. Externally it has been given for tonsillitis, mouth inflammation, sores, and conjunctivitis.

EVIDENCE
Some animal experiments and studies of human tissue indicate that leaf extract does affect the uterus, but the situation is not clear. Consequently, it should not be used during pregnancy and labour unless under medical supervision.

It has also been suggested that it should not be employed for eye infections, including conjunctivitis. The herb is not supported in Germany.

Red clover *Trifolium pratense*

Family Leguminosae/Fabaceae

ORIGIN AND CULTIVATION

The plant originated in Europe and Asia but is now naturalized in North America and Australia. It is of great importance in agriculture as a nitrogen fixer and for making hay.

PLANT DESCRIPTION

Red clover is a biennial or perennial herb growing to a height of about 40 cm (16 in). The leaves consist of three, sometimes four, leaflets with white markings, and the flowering tops are pink to purple.

The parts used in herbal medicine are the flowering tops.

CULINARY AND NUTRITIONAL VALUE

It may have been used as a natural source of food flavouring, but only in very small quantities.

CLAIMS AND FOLKLORE

Red clover extracts have been used as an alterative, to treat skin diseases (particularly eczema and psoriasis), as an expectorant, and to assist with spasmodic coughs.

EVIDENCE

Substances found in red clover include coumarins, isoflavonoids, flavonoids, and saponins. There seems to be little scientific support for the traditional uses of the herb. Animal investigations have shown that the isoflavonoids have oestrogenic properties and, for this reason, should not be used during pregnancy and lactation. Red clover has been included in discredited 'cancer cures'. More recently one of the isoflavonoids has been shown, in animal experiments, to inhibit carcinogenic activity in cell culture.

Rose hip *Rosa canina and other species*

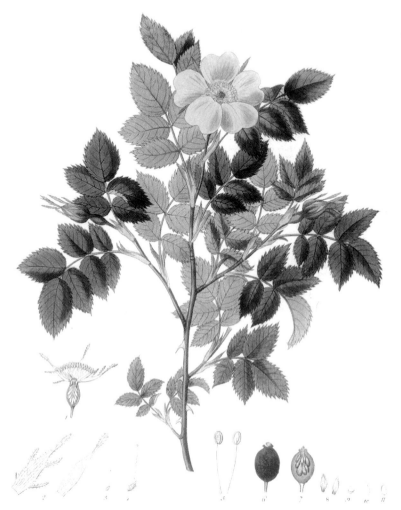

Family Rosaceae

ORIGIN AND CULTIVATION
Some rose species, e.g. *Rosa canina*, are wild in Europe and found in hedgerows, and many rose varieties (cultivars) are famous in horticulture.

PLANT DESCRIPTION
The wild roses are shrubs with long erect, up to 3 m (10 ft), or arching prickly stems. Their flowers are pink or white, giving rise to red or black fruits, which are the 'hips'. The cultivated roses have flowers of varying colours.

CULINARY AND NUTRITIONAL VALUE
The hips can be used to make jellies, preserves, and sauces. Rose hip products (e.g. syrup) are widely included in natural vitamin supplements because they are an excellent source of vitamin C: fresh hips contain 0.5–1.7% of the vitamin, although a significant amount is destroyed during drying and processing. This is supplemented with added vitamin C.

Rose oil (attar of rose) is obtained by distillation from rose petals (*R. damascena* and *R. centifolia* are examples of species cultivated for this purpose). Rose water is the aqueous portion of the distillate after the oil is removed. Rose oil production is very expensive so use is now made of synthetics. The oil and water are used in pharmaceutical products such as perfumes, creams, and soaps. Rose water can be included in jellies and confectionery (e.g. Turkish Delight).

CLAIMS AND FOLKLORE
Extracts of the rose petals and hips are now little used in herbal medicine, but have been employed as a mild treatment for diarrhoea and as a mild diuretic. The essential oil is utilized in aromatherapy for its mildly sedative, antidepressant, and anti-inflammatory properties. In Germany, extracts of *R. gallica* flowers are used to treat mild inflammation of the mouth. Rose hips are not approved in Germany but rose flowers are.

EVIDENCE
It has not been possible to find any scientific investigations relating to rose.

Rue *Ruta graveolens*

Family Rutaceae

ORIGIN AND CULTIVATION

Rue is a native of the Mediterranean region and found growing in poor soil. It is now widely cultivated in temperate regions, including North America, both as a herbal plant and an ornamental.

PLANT DESCRIPTION

It is an evergreen or semi-evergreen shrub growing to a height of 60 cm (2 ft). The leaves are divided and the small yellow flowers give rise to four-lobed capsules. Rue is an aromatic plant with a strong smell.

   The aerial parts are used for herbal medicine.

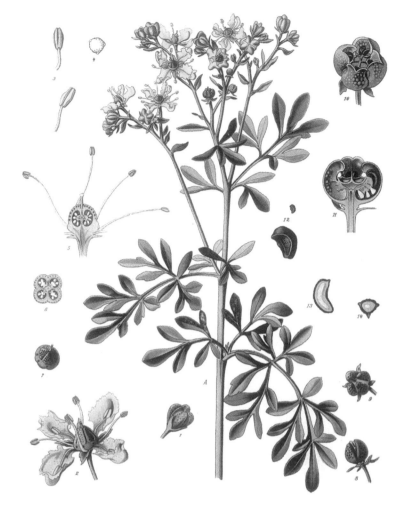

CULINARY AND NUTRITIONAL VALUE

The leaves and oil are used in many beverages, e.g. Vermouth, bitters, Italian grape spirit (grappa), and old-fashioned mead (sack). The oil has been used as a fragrance ingredient in cosmetics such as soaps, creams, and lotions.

CLAIMS AND FOLKLORE

No doubt because of its disagreeable odour, posies of rue and other herbs were once placed in courtrooms to ward off 'jail fever'.

   Extracts have been used externally to deal with sore eyes, eyestrain, and as an insect repellent. Internally the herb has been employed as an antispasmodic (to relieve stomach cramps), for menstrual problems, as a sedative, and an abortifacient. It has been used in homeopathy.

EVIDENCE

Rue contains a number of active principles – flavonoids, alkaloids (quinoline), coumarins, and essential oil.

   Rutin, a flavonoid, has been credited with decreasing blood capillary permeability and fragility. This is possibly concerned with its eye action. The alkaloids and coumarins have antispasmodic action, as shown by some animal experiments.

   Considerable caution should be exercised in the use of rue. The oil or fresh leaves applied to the skin can cause blistering after contact and exposure to sunlight. Taken internally, the oil can cause severe stomach pain, vomiting, and convulsions, and may possibly be fatal. The alkaloid content can act as an abortifacient; therefore, rue should not be taken during pregnancy.

   As there are so many difficulties with rue, the authorities in Germany do not recommend the use of the herb.

137

Sage *Salvia officinalis*

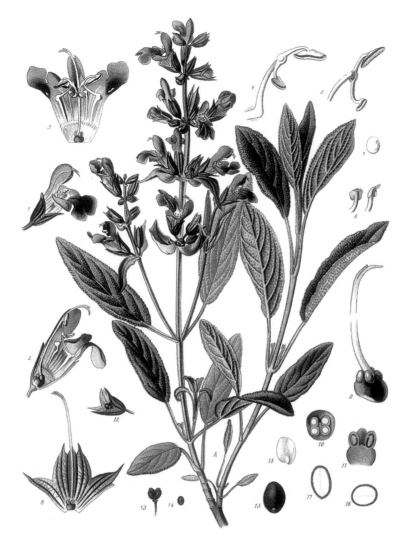

Family Labiatae/Lamiaceae

ORIGIN AND CULTIVATION

Salvia officinalis is a native of the north Mediterranean coast and naturalized in southern Europe. It is said to have been introduced into North America in the seventeenth century and is now cultivated in many countries. As a medicinal herb it was known to the ancient Egyptians, Romans, and Greeks. There are many species and cultivars (varieties) of *Salvia*, often grown as ornamental plants.

S. miltiorhiza is red sage or dan shen, an important Chinese medical herb (known since 206 BC), and also of culinary use. Other *Salvia* species are of value both for culinary and medical use. *S. fruticosa* (*S. triloba*) is Greek sage; *S. lavandulifolia* is narrow-leaved sage or Spanish sage; *S. sclarea* is clary; *S. pomifera* is apple-bearing sage.

PLANT DESCRIPTION

S. officinalis is a perennial with trailing or erect stems up to 45 cm (18 in) long. Its opposite leaves are oblong-ovate to lanceolate and the white, bluish, or reddish flowers are two-lipped.

The leaves and oil are employed in herbal medicine.

CULINARY AND NUTRITIONAL VALUE

The fresh or dried herb is used for stuffings (e.g. sage and onion with goose), and in cheese, meats, sausages, and beverages. The commercially available product is normally a mixture of species. Essential oil produced from sage is used in the food and pharmaceutical industries.

CLAIMS AND FOLKLORE

As stated earlier, *S. officinalis* has a long history of medical use. Extracts taken internally have been recommended for anxiety, insomnia, and problems of digestion; it has been employed externally for insect bites and various infections (throat, mouth, skin).

Red sage (dan shen) root is recommended for heart and circulatory problems.

EVIDENCE

There seems to be support for the traditional uses of sage extract. These appear to be related to the essential oil (its major constituent is thujone), which, like many other essential oils, is carminative, antiseptic, and antispasmodic. However, the oil is toxic if ingested directly, and sage herbal medicine should not be taken during pregnancy and lactation. It is probably a good idea not to use the herb over a prolonged period.

Sage oil can be a skin irritant and consequently is not suitable for aromatherapy. The herb is approved in Germany.

Saw palmetto *Serenoa repens syn. S. serrulata*

Family Palmae/Arecaceae

ORIGIN AND CULTIVATION

Saw palmetto forms dense thickets in the coastal areas of southeastern North America; the berries are harvested mainly in central and southern Florida and southern Georgia.

PLANT DESCRIPTION

It is a palm growing to a height of 2–4 m (16 ft) with blue–green to yellow–green palmate leaves, 45–100 cm (3 ft) wide. The tiny cream flowers give rise to blue–black fruits or berries of olive-like shape, 2.5 cm (1 in) in length.

Its fresh or dried berries are the source of herbal medicine.

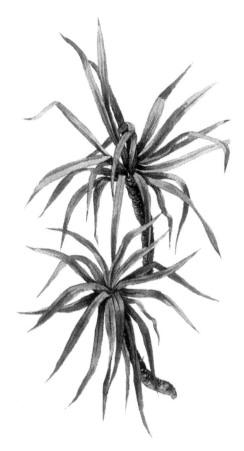

FOOD AND NUTRITIONAL VALUE

The berries were eaten by the native North Americans and considered nutritious.

CLAIMS AND FOLKLORE

Saw palmetto has been used in herbal medicine for a number of reasons, for example as a diuretic, and an expectorant for bronchial and catarrhal problems. Modern interest mainly concerns its effect on the male reproductive system, and various properties have been attributed to it; for instance, it is said to be useful in dealing with problems associated with a non-malignant enlargement of the prostate gland, and impotence; it is also used as an aphrodisiac in men. In women, it has sometimes been claimed to be effective for breast enlargement.

EVIDENCE

Among the chemical substances present in saw palmetto are steroids (beta-sitosterol), fixed oils, essential oils, and flavonoids.

There have been numerous human and animal investigations. In Germany, the drug is supported for relieving micturition (desire to urinate) in certain stages of non-malignant prostate enlargement, although it does not seem to reduce the actual enlargement. It has also been pointed out that only the fat-soluble components of the drug are active, so that a tea with only water-soluble components is not effective. Part of the scientific explanation of the action of the drug could be that it inhibits a very large percentage of the activity of the enzyme prostate 5-α-reductase, which is involved in the size increase of the prostate.

Because of the reported hormone-like (anti-androgen and oestrogen) activities of the drug, it may interfere with existing hormone therapy (oral contraceptive and hormone replacement). Its use during pregnancy and lactation should be avoided – indeed any employment of the drug should first be discussed with a medical advisor.

Senna (Alexandrian and Khartoum) *Cassia senna;* senna (tinnevelly and Indian) *Cassia angustifolia*

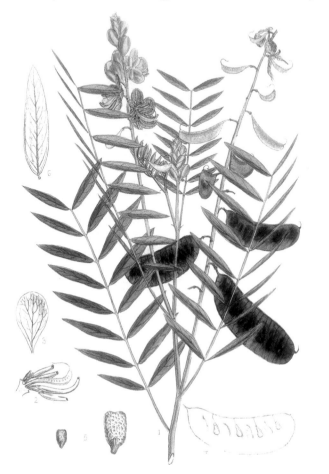

Family Leguminosae/Fabaceae

ORIGIN AND CULTIVATION
Cassia senna is native, and cultivated, in areas such as Arabia, Somalia, and Sudan. *C. angustifolia* is found in the Indian subcontinent and cultivated mainly in southern and northern India, and Pakistan.

PLANT DESCRIPTION
Both species are small shrubs up to 1 m (3 ft) in height, with divided leaves. The yellow flowers give rise to pods (fruits), about 7 cm (3 in) in length.

The pods and leaves constitute the herbal drug.

CULINARY AND NUTRITIONAL VALUE
None.

CLAIMS AND FOLKLORE
Senna pods and leaves are well known for their laxative properties. The drug was introduced into Europe in the ninth and tenth centuries by Arabian physicians.

The chemical constitution of the pods and leaves has been well investigated. It is normally agreed that the active principles are anthraquinones – A and B sennosides. Their action leads to a stimulation of the colon, although the exact mechanism is not fully understood. A soft stool is the result of senna action. Senna on its own can cause griping pains and colic; consequently preparations are usually mixed with other herbs.

A number of related species have been used to treat other ailments, such as ringworm, venereal disease, and various bacterial and fungal infections.

EVIDENCE
It is well accepted that senna is an effective laxative, but care should be taken with preparations; they are best standardized to sennoside B. The drug should not be given to patients with intestinal obstruction or undiagnosed abdominal symptoms. Standardized preparations might possibly be tolerated during pregnancy and lactation.

As with all laxatives, it is best not to use senna over a prolonged period. The drug is supported in Germany.

Senna should not be confused with the spice 'cassia' – a species of *Cinnamomum*.

Sesame, beniseed, til *Sesamum indicum*

Family Pedaliaceae

ORIGIN AND CULTIVATION

Sesame originated in Africa and, early on, was taken to India. Today it is cultivated in China, India, Africa, the USA, and Central and South America. It is one of the most ancient of oilseeds.

PLANT DESCRIPTION

The plant is an annual with white, pink, or purplish flowers. The seeds can be white, yellow, grey, red, brown, or black in colour. They are sometimes marketed without hulls (seed coats) and the kernels are white. The seeds are about 4 mm (0.15 in) in length.

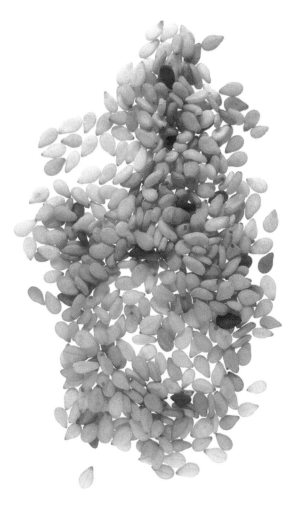

CULINARY AND NUTRITIONAL VALUE

Seeds and kernels are utilized in food in many ways. They can be included in soup, porridge, sweetmeats, and nut snacks, and sprinkled over cakes, bread, and pastries. Products containing sesame seeds including 'tahini', 'halvah', and 'niu bi tang'.

Sesame seeds are an important source of oil used in the manufacture of margarine, cooking fats, soaps, paints, and as a lubricant and illuminant. The oil is highly unsaturated (oleic and linoleic acids predominate), and rarely becomes rancid because of the presence of phenolic substances. In India it is used as a substitute for 'ghee', and in perfumery.

The seed may contain up to 60% oil and 20–5% protein, and is a good source of calcium, phosphorus, iron, and B and E vitamins. There may be a little carotene. The fibre content is reasonable.

Sesame seed is almost free of antinutritional factors but does contain oxalates in the seed coat, although this is not usually a problem. The substantial amount of phosphorus present is tied up in phytic acid or phytin, and this decreases the bioavailability of minerals such as calcium and iron.

Some people are highly sensitive to sesame seed.

CLAIMS AND FOLKLORE

Sesame seeds have been used in herbal medicine for a variety of ailments, including dizziness and blurred vision, and as a laxative.

EVIDENCE

There seems to be no organized research to support any claims.

Skullcap, scullcap *Scutellaria lateriflora*

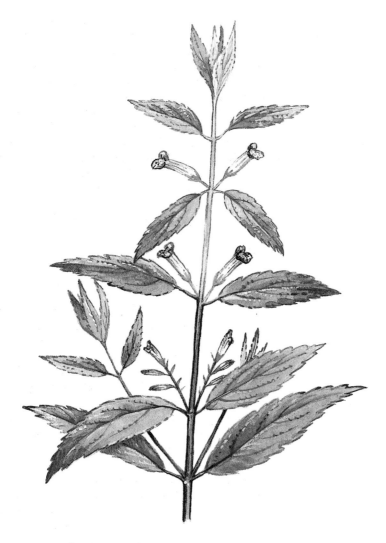

Family Labiatae/Lamiaceae

ORIGIN AND CULTIVATION

Skullcap grows wild in the USA and Canada, and is found in damp conditions on riverbanks and in moist woods. Other *Scutellaria* species used in herbal medicine are *S. baicalensis* (Chinese medicine) and *S. galericulata* (Europe).

PLANT DESCRIPTION

The plant is a perennial growing to a height of 60 cm (2 ft), with pink to blue flowers giving rise to fruits, which have been likened to skullcaps.

Its aerial parts are used to prepare herbal medicine.

CULINARY AND NUTRITIONAL VALUE

None.

CLAIMS AND FOLKLORE

It was used by some North American natives for menstrual problems. At one time it was a treatment for rabies. Modern herbalists may recommend it for nervous complaints – its reputed antispasmodic activity may deal with muscular tension caused by stress and worry.

EVIDENCE

Skullcap contains flavonoids, iridoids, essential oils, and tannins.

There seem to have been few scientific investigations into the therapeutic value of *S. lateriflora*. Although some herbalists still recommend the drug, serious doubts have been raised about its efficacy. Some reports state that it can damage the liver, although this may relate to an adulterant, namely germander (genus *Teucrium*). Because of this situation, a number of modern authorities do not recommend use of the herb, and it definitely should not be taken during pregnancy and lactation.

Slimming products

There is a simple statement that sums up the situation regarding weight gain. If you take in, in food and drink, more energy than you use up in maintaining vital body processes and daily activity, you will gain weight. Therefore, in order to lose weight you need to shift the balance, either by eating and drinking less or by increasing activity, so that energy used is greater than what you consume. This sounds simple – but the fact that obesity and overweight are rising markedly in most countries in the world shows us that it is not.

The recommended way of losing weight is to attack both sides of the equation, i.e. by increasing activity and by reducing energy intake. Without an increase in activity very low intakes of energy from food may be needed, and at energy intakes below about 1200 kcal per day it becomes difficult to ensure that the diet supplies all the essential vitamins and minerals. Today it is usually recommended that people control their intake, to a level of about 500 kcal below their energy needs. So the average woman who needs a little less than 2000 kcal to maintain weight should get about 1500 per day. She will then lose weight at about 0.5-1 kg per week, and ensure that she is losing the majority of the weight from her fat stores. Rapid weight loss results in loss of lean tissue, and as this is the most active tissue, which uses up most energy, loss of lean tissue causes a reduction of energy needs in the long term; this means it is easier to put the weight back on again.

Energy intake can be controlled by a variety of means, but it is usually recommended that individuals restrict fat and fatty foods while eating plenty of fruit and vegetables, reasonable amounts of starchy carbohydrates, preferably wholegrain, and moderate quantities of protein foods such as lean meat, fish, pulses, and dairy products. It is important to ensure that food sources of both calcium and iron are adequate, especially for women.

Because of the difficulties people have in losing weight, there is a huge market for slimming aids, which either attempt to reduce energy intake or purport to increase metabolic rate and use up more energy. These are discussed below.

MEAL REPLACEMENTS

These products are intended to replace one or more meals per day to ensure a controlled low energy intake. They may take the form of milky drinks, either ready to drink or as powders to mix with skimmed milk, or as cereal or confectionery-type bars. It is usually recommended that two to three drinks or bars are taken each day as a replacement for meals and snacks, and that a balanced, low energy meal, is taken for the third meal such that a total daily energy intake of about 1200 kcal is supplied. Commonly, each drink or bar provides about 200 kcal and a range of nutrients, such that the majority of the day's requirements for all known nutrients are covered. Most have a significant amount of dietary fibre or non-starch polysaccharides, which, it is suggested, aid satiety.

These products have, in the past, been frowned upon by some nutritionists and dietitians as they do not help people to learn how to eat healthily and control energy intake. However, it is now recognized that they may be useful for some people who find it difficult to regulate energy intake using ordinary food. They provide a controlled energy meal, ensuring a good range of essential nutrients. They remove the temptations involved in shopping for food and cooking meals, and as they are so different from the normal diet may serve to remind people that they are controlling their weight.

The main drawback is that, if used inappropriately, low-calorie meal replacements may result in very rapid weight loss. Recommended energy intakes for weight-reducing programmes should be designed to allow the individual to lose weight gradually. Heavier people will lose weight at higher energy intakes than lighter people. Therefore, if someone who is initially very overweight or obese follows a 1200 kcal regimen they will lose weight far too quickly and lose more lean tissue. This makes it easier for them to gain weight, and harder to lose it again in the future. It is therefore advisable for such people to get advice from a dietitian or doctor before embarking on such diets.

PRODUCTS THAT BIND FAT AND REDUCE ABSORPTION

Fat in foods has the highest amount of energy, weight-for-weight. There is a range of products for sale that contain substances that are said to bind fat in the digestive tract, preventing its absorption and thereby leading to weight loss.

Galactomannan/glucomannan

These non-starch polysaccharide supplements are advocated as aids to weight loss due to their ability to reduce fat absorption, thus reducing the energy available from the meal. They are also recommended for their supposed ability to swell up in the stomach and cause early satiety. It is suggested that they be consumed with water before a meal, and that they will then prevent overeating. There is some scientific basis for each of these suggestions, but evidence for their effectiveness as slimming aids is not convincing. The dose of viscous polysaccharide needed to show effects is quite large, e.g. 10 g or more per meal, and doses as high as this are rarely recommended because gastrointestinal side-effects, such as excess wind causing bloating and discomfort, can be marked. If presented in capsule form the materials may not dissolve or swell in the stomach, and will therefore not have the desired effect.

Other plant polysaccharides

These often appear as ingredients in multiple-ingredient weight loss supplements (see below). They may simply be called non-starch polysaccharides or heteropolysaccharides, or may be given precise names (e.g. glucomannan). Evidence for the effectiveness of these in the amounts usually recommended is rarely forthcoming.

Chitin and chitosan

Sometimes called 'fat magnets'. Chitin and chitosan are derived from the shells of crabs, shrimps, and other shellfish. Chitin is a long-chain polysaccharide with a similar structure to some of the plant polysaccharides, and is sometimes erroneously referred to as a dietary fibre supplement. It has been shown in some experiments (mostly in animal studies) to bind dietary fat, cholesterol, and bile salts in the intestine. It is therefore sold as a supplement for weight loss and to reduce blood cholesterol levels.

There is some evidence for the effectiveness of chitin as a cholesterol-lowering agent and as an aid to weight loss in human studies, but more research is needed to confirm doses needed and side-effects, e.g. on fat-soluble vitamin absorption. Gastrointestinal side-effects may occur at high (i.e. effective) doses, and chitin should not be consumed by people with an allergy to shellfish.

PRODUCTS THAT CLAIM TO INCREASE METABOLIC RATE

These are usually products that contain mixtures of ingredients that are alleged to increase metabolic rate and therefore 'burn-off' fat. Ingredient lists often include substances that do have some role in the metabolism of fat or energy, but rarely has the compound multi-ingredient product itself been scientifically demonstrated to either increase metabolic rate or induce weight loss.

Examples of ingredients found in such products might be: chromium salts, cayenne pepper, grapeseed extract, caffeine, L-carnitine, B vitamins, hydroxycitric acid, *Garcinia cambogia*, ginseng, astragalus, reishi mushroom, guarana (which is high in caffeine), cider vinegar, and many others.

Some of these products may contain pharmacologically active ingredients, and indeed may have effects on the nervous system such that the vendors warn about side-effects such as dry mouth, nausea, bloating, and feeling 'heady' or dizzy. The evidence for their effectiveness in aiding weight loss is anecdotal, and such products are not recommended for pregnant or nursing mothers, or people with medical conditions such as diabetes or thyroid problems. It would be wise to consult a qualified medical practitioner before taking such supplements.

Slippery elm *Ulmus rubra syn. U. fulva*

Family Ulmaceae

ORIGIN AND CULTIVATION
The plant is native to eastern Canada and eastern and central USA. It is most common in the Appalachian mountains. Other species are also used, e.g. white elm (*Ulmus americana*).

PLANT DESCRIPTION
Slippery elm is a large tree growing to a height of 20 m (65 ft). Its obovate hairy leaves are up to 20 cm (8 in) in length. The small reddish flowers give rise to winged fruits.

Herbal medicine is made from the inner bark of the trunk and branches of the tree.

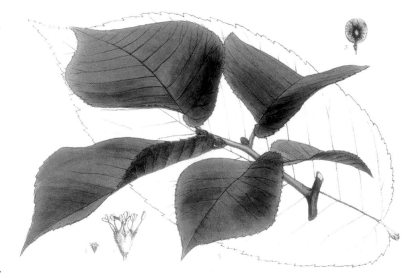

CULINARY AND NUTRITIONAL VALUE
It has been suggested that slippery elm is not suitable as a flavouring agent in foods, although it has been recommended as a nutritious food for convalescents and babies.

CLAIMS AND FOLKLORE
White elm was utilized by native North Americans, and the bark of European *Ulmus* species was used by Dioscorides (first century).

Extracts of slippery elm, being soothing and protective (demulcent and emollient) to surface (skin and intestinal) body tissues, are given internally for conditions such as bronchitis, coughs, gastric and duodenal ulcers, colitis, and other digestive problems. Externally, it has been employed for various skin conditions such as wounds, burns, and boils, and in poultices for drawing out splinters.

EVIDENCE
Extracts of the outer bark can act as an abortifacient and therefore only the inner bark is used in herbal medicine.

The inner bark contains carbohydrates, particularly mucilage, which is the soothing principle of the medicine. Tannins are also present.

Slippery elm is generally regarded as non-toxic.

Soya bean, soybean *Glycine max*

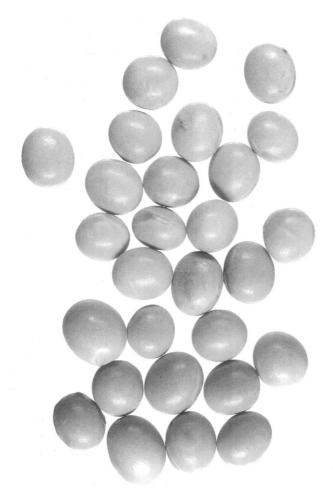

Family Leguminosae/Fabaceae

ORIGIN AND CULTIVATION

Soya bean was first domesticated in northeastern China in about the eleventh century BC. From there the crop spread to Manchuria, Korea, Japan, and Russia, and to other Asian countries. It was introduced into the USA at the beginning of the twentieth century as a hay or pasture crop, but became cultivated for oilseeds and is now the most important cash crop in that country. Soya bean is one of the world's great oilseed plants.

The major world producers of seed are the USA, Brazil, China, and Argentina, but it is grown in some Asian countries, often by smallholders. Soya bean is a subtropical plant and is cultivated throughout the middle latitudes of the world. It is not suitable for the UK.

PLANT DESCRIPTION

The plant is an annual growing to a height of 20–180 cm (70 in), with white or lilac flowers and pods containing two to three seeds (yellow, green, brown, or black). Soya seeds are 4–8 mm (0.15–0.30 in) in diameter.

CULINARY AND NUTRITIONAL VALUE

Most of the seed yield (90%) is used for oil production. The seed oil is included in cooking oil, salad oil, margarine, and shortening, and there are some industrial uses. Meal, after oil extraction, is a popular constituent of animal food.

Soya beans, whole or split, may be cooked as a vegetable, but most seed to be used for human food is processed to form products, some of which have been known in the East for centuries and are now quite well known in Western countries.

- Soya milk: made by adding water to defatted soya bean meal together with some sugar and refined soya oil. It is manufactured by traditional and industrial methods. As the milk is free of lactose, it is suitable for lactose intolerant people – and those suffering from allergies to cow's milk, eggs, and wheat. Soya milk can be prepared with the minimum of time and expense by relatively simple methods of technology anywhere in the world.

- 'Tempeh': sometimes described as a soya cheese. It is estimated that 50% of the Indonesian population consume a daily average of 18 g of tempeh as a meat substitute. This is cooked by steaming, boiling, or frying, and is included in meals that may contain rice and vegetables. It only commands one-fifth to one-third of the price of beef or buffalo meat. Tempeh is manufactured by a fermentation process involving the fungal mould *Rhizopus*.

- 'Tofu': sometimes described as soya bean curd. Soya milk is coagulated with a calcium or magnesium salt, the whey is discarded, and the curds are pressed to form

Soya bean, soybean

a cohesive product that can be puréed for dressings, dips, and spreads, or eaten separately.

- 'Miso': soya beans, mixed with rice and barley, are fermented with the fungal mould *Aspergillus oryzae* (or *A. sojae*) to give a product that is blended, mashed, and pasteurized, and known as 'miso'.

- 'Natto': this is another fermented soya product (the fermenting organism is *Bacillus natto*). The product can, for example, be used as a topping for rice, added to 'miso' soup, or sautéed with vegetables; it is also used as an hors d'oeuvre.

- Soya sauce: this dark liquid substance is well known in the East and to those in the West who enjoy Eastern cuisine – it is also a constituent of some Western sauces. Again, it is a fermentation product. Traditionally, it takes a year to prepare but it can be manufactured in 24 hours by a chemical process.

Fermentation serves a number of useful functions. Soya (and some other legumes) is difficult to digest and can give rise to flatulence (due to the oligosaccharides stachyose and raffinose); fermentation reduces this problem. Also, soya contains a number of antinutritional factors, in particular an antitrypsin factor that reduces the efficiency of the human protein digesting enzyme trypsin. Again, fermentation improves the situation.

Other food products made from soya include flour, grits, protein concentrates, isolates, extenders, and extruded substances, which are used in a vast array of foods, including bakery and meat products. 'Soynuts' are also available. Where heat is involved in the production of these materials it will reduce the antinutritional factors. Soya-protein isolates avoid flatulence problems. There is now much debate about the safety of genetically modified soya. As soya is found in so many food products, and as the genetically modified and normal seeds are often mixed after harvest, there is indeed a problem, but products containing soya may be labelled as free of genetically modified seeds. Spun soya protein resembles in some ways the muscle fibres of meat, which therefore makes it useful in products (analogues) that are imitations of meat.

There is variation concerning the chemical constituents of soya bean. Oil content varies between 15% and 24%, with an average of 19%; protein, content is 30–50%, with an average of 35%, which is better than most other legumes. The oil is highly unsaturated, with 25% oleic acid (monounsaturated) and 50% linoleic acid (polyunsaturated), although the fatty acid composition of the oil may change with new varieties (cultivars). Soya protein has a well balanced amino acid composition, although, as in other legumes, low methionine and cysteine are the limiting amino acids, but this is not a problem if the soya is complemented with cereal protein; or, if the total amount of food consumed provides the energy required, there is usually more protein than is needed, and so there are adequate quantities of even the limiting amino acid.

Soya flours, grits, concentrates, and isolates contain 50–90% protein, highly digestible and much more than toasted and steamed whole beans contain. Other soya products have reasonable amounts of protein: tofu, 8%; tempeh, 17%; miso, 12%; natto, 11%; soya milk, 3%; and soya sauce, 6%. Oil quantities vary: tofu, 5%; tempeh, 8%; natto 7%; miso, 5%; various soya flours from defatted, 1%, to full fat, 20%; isolates, 0.1%; soya milk, 2%; and soya sauce, 1%.

As regards vitamins, whole soya beans contain a little carotene, some E, and the B complex. In general terms, these vitamins are found in soya products. As stated earlier in the book, vitamin B_{12} is not found in plant foods; however, it has been reported in soya products. This could be the result of bacterial contamination, or it could be an 'analogue' of B_{12}, which is not biologically active – a similar situation occurs in the algae (see p. 2). Vitamin C does not occur in soya or its products, except sprouts (germinated seeds).

Soya can be a good source of calcium, iron, zinc, phosphorus, and magnesium, although the phytin or phytate (calcium and magnesium salt of a phosphorus compound) present may affect the absorption of iron, but vitamin C in a diet may enhance this absorption. Calcium content of soya milk and tofu is somewhat variable – it depends on the commercial brand and, of course, calcium salt is a coagulant in the manufacture of tofu. It has been stated that calcium absorption from soya in women is about 80% of that from cow's milk, and therefore soya milk may be supplemented with calcium. A view that has been put forward is that zinc absorption from soya by vegetarians is possibly inadequate.

Soya and most of its products are a good source of dietary fibre, but this is low in tofu and soya milk.

It is clear that soya beans are an important food source. There are a number of reasons for this: the plant can grown in a variety of soils and under a wide range of climatic conditions, the edible protein yield per unit area is one of the highest of all plant sources, and, as previously stated, soya protein is very good from a nutritional point of view.

Sterols (see p. 105) are found in soya, and it is the best commercial source of lecithin (see p. 98).

Soya bean, soybean

CLAIMS AND FOLKLORE

Soya is often regarded as one of the best anticancer foods. Populations consuming Soya regularly are said to have lower levels of breast cancer in females and prostate cancer in males, less osteoporosis and fewer menopausal symptoms. Soya consumption is also said to combat cardiovascular disease and improve gastrointestinal health.

Its fibre has a modest beneficial effect on blood glucose levels in diabetics, and can lower total and low-density lipoprotein cholesterol. Soya-protein isolate also lowers blood cholesterol.

EVIDENCE

Medical claims for soya are based on human studies, animal experiments, and epidemiological evidence. Soya contains isoflavones (flavonoids), such as genistein, daidzein, and glycetein, known as phytoestrogens, which are similar to human body oestrogens. These isoflavones, if consumed by women, reduce the level of blood oestrogen, one of the risk factors in breast cancer. Also, consumption of soya and its products is 10 times greater in Asian cultures than in Western countries. Breast and prostate cancer is considerably greater in Western countries than in the East. Although not direct evidence, these comparisons do provide some support for the value of soya as regards some types of cancer.

The tolerance to soya is good, although there has been some reservation about the exposure of infants to soya-based diets because of the isoflavones.

In 1999 the US Food and Drug Administration authorized the use of health claims in food labelling regarding the role of soya protein in reducing the risk of coronary heart disease, although there is some controversy about its effect in this respect. The decision was based on the Food and Drug Administration's conclusion that including foods containing soya protein in a diet low in saturated fat and cholesterol may reduce the risk of coronary heart disease by lowering blood cholesterol levels. The following is an example of the type of claim allowed:

> Diets low in saturated fat and cholesterol that include 25 grams of soy (soya) protein a day may reduce the risk of heart disease. One serving of (name of food) provides x grams of soy (soya) protein.

In 2002 the UK Joint Health Claims Initiative followed suit allowing a generic claim:

> The inclusion of at least 25 g soya protein per day as part of a diet low in saturated fat can help reduce blood cholesterol

with the proviso that any product for which a claim was made should contain at least 5g of soya protein per portion.

Sports supplements

PROTEIN SUPPLEMENTS

Various types of protein supplements are available. They are usually sold as a means of increasing muscle bulk, sometimes as protein powders alone, sometimes with added carbohydrate. Some research supports the anabolic (muscle-building) effects of consuming about 2.0–2.5 g of protein per kilogram of body weight each day during resistance training by athletes who compete in strength/power events. However, because they have relatively high energy requirements, eating a balanced diet usually supplies all the protein they need. There is no conclusive evidence to suggest that taking protein supplements will enhance muscle mass in athletes who are eating well and doing high-quality resistance training.

WHEY PROTEIN

This particular type of protein is a by-product of the cheese-making industry. The liquid left after the cheese curd is separated contains protein, which, it has been suggested, has a high biological value (i.e. it is a relatively 'complete' protein and is easily used by the body) and promotes gains in muscle mass greater than other protein supplements. The studies demonstrating that whey protein builds muscle have mostly been done in animals. Evidence for any effect on performance related to muscle building in humans is limited.

Another proposed positive effect of consumption of whey protein is that it may enhance immune function. It is suggested that, because whey contains significant amounts of the amino acid cysteine, it promotes the production of an antioxidant, glutathione, which is necessary for development of the immune response. There is not a lot of scientific evidence for this, and again most studies have been done in animals, but one study showed an increase in peak power, 30-second work capacity, and glutathione levels when 18 athletes were supplemented with 20 g of whey protein per day. The authors suggest that the whey protein reduced oxidative stress and muscle fatigue.

Not all whey protein is the same. Different methods of processing affect the amount and nature of the protein. Whey protein hydrolysate is considered inferior, as the protein is denatured by heat processing during preparation. Whey protein isolate (the most expensive type) contains most protein (about 90 g per 100 g), whereas whey protein concentrate contains less than half this (35 g per 100 g). Whey protein prepared using ion-exchange filtration appears to retain most of the supposed immuno-enhancing components. Thus, those wishing to gain the proposed immune system benefits should choose whey isolates prepared by ion-exchange filtration.

CHROMIUM

Chromium is a trace element that is involved in insulin action and maintaining blood sugar levels. Athletes appear to have increased urinary excretion of the mineral compared with sedentary adults. Chromium, usually as chromium picolinate, which is easily absorbed, is taken by some athletes in the belief that it will increase strength. Scientific evidence for this is equivocal.

CREATINE

This is a naturally occurring amino acid (methyl-guanidine acetic acid) found in skeletal muscles. It is made in the body from other amino acids, but is also present in meat. The average adult daily requirement is thought to be about 2 g; about 1 g of this is supplied by the diet in meat-eaters, but must be produced endogenously by vegetarians. In muscle, in the form of creatine phosphate, creatine provides a source of fuel for sprints or high-intensity exercise lasting up to 10 seconds.

Creatine monohydrate is the most common dietary supplement and it has been shown that large doses will increase muscle creatine and creatine phosphate. The response to creatine supplementation is variable, and about 30% of people will not show increased levels sufficient to improve performance, possibly because the levels in muscle were high to begin with. Creatine supplementation has been shown to enhance performance in exercise involving repeated sprints or bouts of high-intensity exercise followed by short recovery intervals. It has also been shown in some studies to increase strength. Athletes taking this supplement will be given a loading protocol (e.g. four doses of 5 g daily for 5 days, or 3 g per day for up to 28 days), whereby the muscle levels are built up to saturation, followed by a daily small dose to maintain levels. Some studies suggest that carbohydrate taken with the creatine will enhance uptake into muscles. No long-term studies of creatine supplementation have been reported but as yet no adverse effects have been described.

GLUTAMINE

This is an amino acid that acts as fuel for the immune system. Athletes who are training hard have been shown to have low circulating levels of glutamine in the hours after hard exercise.

Although exercise is generally beneficial to health, it has been suggested that athletes in heavy training, or who have recently completed an endurance event, are more susceptible to infections than sedentary people. It is possible that severe exercise results in a temporary reduction in the body's immune response. It has been proposed that the

Sports supplements

reduction in circulating glutamine may result in a reduced ability to mount an immune response to opportunistic infections. Experimental work investigating the idea that glutamine supplements may protect athletes from infections has not yet been conclusive. However, the supplements are sold widely and research is ongoing.

SPORTS DRINKS

These are drinks that are designed to enable athletes to replace fluid lost during exercise. Dehydration can affect athletic performance, especially in endurance exercise such as long-distance running, but also in sports such as football or tennis where there is intermittent high-intensity exercise.

Sports drinks usually contain sugars (often as glucose) and electrolytes (sodium and potassium), but may also contain other substances such as choline and glycerol. They are designed with specific concentrations of glucose and electrolytes that are said to allow optimal rates of fluid absorption. The carbohydrate is also a source of energy. Concentrated solutions of carbohydrate can cause gastrointestinal upsets in some people.

Glycerol added to sports drinks has been shown in some studies, but not others, to enhance fluid absorption and prevent fatigue. It may be useful in endurance exercise, especially in hot conditions, but it may cause headaches and nausea, and is not advisable for those with high blood pressure or kidney problems, or for pregnant women.

St John's wort *Hypericum perforatum*

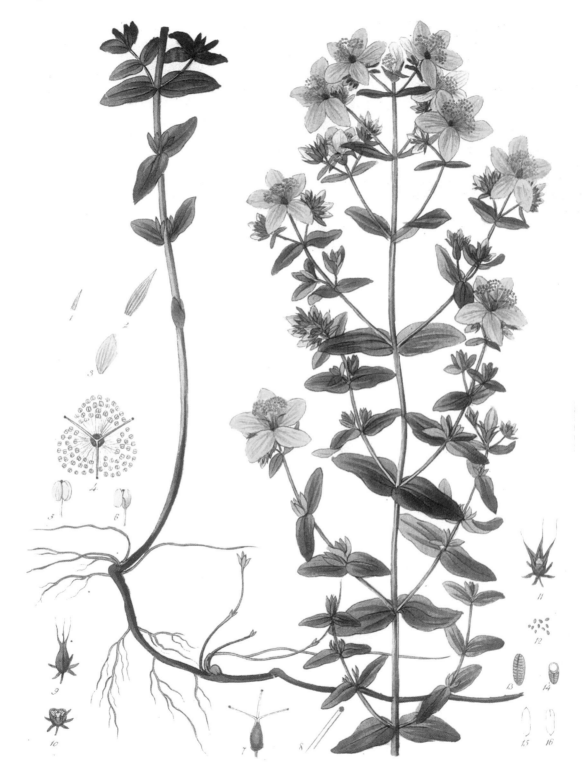

St John's wort

Family Guttiferae/Hypericaceae

ORIGIN AND CULTIVATION

St John's wort is thought to be indigenous to Europe, but is now naturalized in Asia, Africa, North America, and Australia. It grows in waste places, along roadsides, and in woods and hedgerows.

PLANT DESCRIPTION

It is a perennial with linear–ovate leaves 2.5 cm (1 in) long, and growing to a height of 30–60 cm (2 ft). The stem branches at the top and carries yellow flowers 2.5 cm (1 in) wide. Glands are found on the stem, leaves, and flowers. There is a rhizome.

Flowering tops are used to prepare herbal medicine.

CULINARY AND NUTRITIONAL VALUE

Extracts of St John's wort can be added as flavouring to foods (e.g. pastilles and alcoholic beverages) as long as the anthroquinone hypericin does not exceed certain values.

CLAIMS AND FOLKLORE

The herb has been used for hundreds of years in traditional medicine. It has been stated that its alleged magical properties were partly due to the fluorescent red pigment that oozes like blood from crushed flowers.

Taken internally, St John's wort is said to act as a sedative or antidepressant, and could be used to treat ailments such as anxiety, nervous tension, menopausal disturbances, and insomnia. Applied externally, its presumed anti-inflammatory, astringent, antiviral, and antiseptic properties are considered useful in dealing with burns, bruises, and injuries (especially deep or painful wounds involving nerve damage).

In health food shops, St John's wort is found in teas, tinctures, capsules, and tablets; the herb can be soaked in oil and the infusion used to treat skin problems. The herb is found in skin-care cosmetic products.

EVIDENCE

It contains a wide range of chemical constituents. Those particularly implicated in its medical actions are the anthroquinone hypericin (although some doubt has been expressed about this), flavonoids, and tannins.

Animal experiments and human studies support many of the claims made for St John's wort. Indeed, the plant, with its reported antiviral action, is being used in studies of AIDS; also, synthetic hypericin is under development as an antiviral agent for treating transfusion blood supply. A recent medical opinion is that St John's wort might be suitable for treating mild, but not acute, depression.

It is known that cattle, sheep, and other animals may experience photosensitization after eating the plant. Consequently, it might be wise for light-skinned persons to avoid direct sunlight after ingestion.

There have been several reports suggesting that St John's Wort may interact adversely with some prescribed drugs (e.g. anti-depressant drugs; Digoxin). People who are taking prescription drugs are therefore advised to consult a medical practitioner before taking the herb.

St John's wort should not be taken during pregnancy and lactation. Approval is given to the drug in Germany.

Strawberry   *Fragaria vesca, Fragaria × ananassa*

Family Rosaceae

ORIGIN AND CULTIVATION

Fragaria vesca is the wild strawberry, and is found in Europe, Asia, and North America. The cultivated strawberry is *Fragaria × ananassa*, which arose by hybridization in Europe from two imported American species – *F. virginiana* and *F. chiloensis*. There are now many cultivars and cultivation can take place in every continent, although it occurs mainly in the Northern Hemisphere.

PLANT DESCRIPTION

Strawberry is a perennial plant with a crown of trifoliate leaves up to 6 cm (2–3 in) in length. The white flowers give rise to the well known red, juicy fruits, in which are embedded the tiny yellow pips or 'seeds' (botanically speaking, fruits). Vegetative reproduction is carried out by radiating prostrate stems or runners.

The parts used in herbal medicine are the leaves, roots, and fruits.

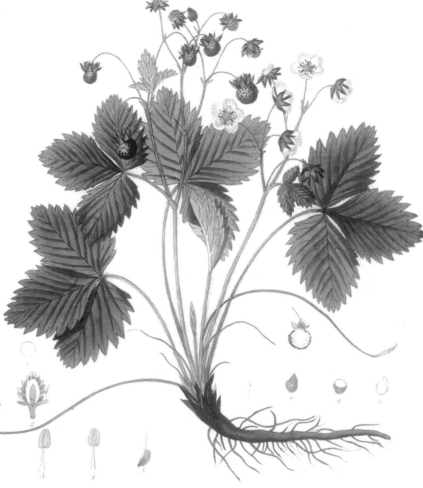

CULINARY AND NUTRITIONAL VALUE

The fruit is utilized for dessert, canning, freezing, jams, jellies, ice-cream, syrups, juices, and bakery products. Its water content is very high (about 90%), the sugars present are mainly glucose and fructose, the percentage of vitamin C present is high (77 mg per 100 g), and the acids in the fruit are essentially citric and malic.

CLAIMS AND FOLKLORE

There does not seem to be much use for strawberry in modern herbalism. The plant has been employed internally for diarrhoea, dysentery, gout, and some other conditions, and externally for skin complaints.

EVIDENCE

Flavonoids, tannins, and an essential oil are found in the leaves. The chemical constitution of the fruit has been stated above.

No scientific investigations related to the herbal value of strawberry have been found. It is not recommended in Germany.

Sumach *Rhus glabra and other species*

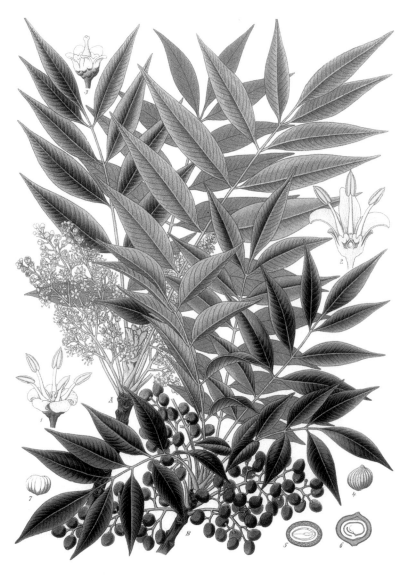

Family Anacardiaceae

ORIGIN AND CULTIVATION
Rhus glabra is the smooth sumach and grows on the borders of woods, hedgerows, and in waste places in North America. Other sumach species of interest are *R. aromatica*, *R. coriaria*, and *R. chinensis*.

R. radicans is poison ivy, well known for causing severe contact dermatitis.

PLANT DESCRIPTION
The plant is a deciduous shrub or tree growing to a height of 3–5 m (16 ft). Its leaves are pinnate and turn brilliant red in September and October. The light red flowers give rise to red berries.

The root bark and berries are used in herbal medicine.

CULINARY AND NUTRITIONAL VALUE
None.

CLAIMS AND FOLKLORE
Sumach has been taken internally for diarrhoea, dysentery, to reduce fever, and for urinary complaints. Externally, it has been used for skin complaints, haemorrhoids, and as a gargle for mouth and throat problems.

EVIDENCE
Sumach is rich in tannins, and the astringent and diuretic properties of these compounds no doubt have been responsible for some of the herbal uses of the plant.

Sunflower seed *Helianthus annuus*

Family Compositae/Asteraceae

ORIGIN AND CULTIVATION

Sunflower probably originated in the southwestern part of North America, and there is evidence of cultivation as early as 900 BC. The seed has been used as food by the North American Indians for thousands of years. It was taken to Europe in the sixteenth century, and by the early nineteenth century became an important oilseed crop in Russia. This is still the case in Russia, and other important countries for cultivation are the USA and Argentina.

PLANT DESCRIPTION

The plant may grow to a height of 3.5 m (11–12 ft), but shorter plants are preferred in cultivation. Its very large yellow flower head, 10–14 cm (6 in) in diameter, is well known. The seeds (botanically speaking, fruits) can be white, brown, black, or striped, and up to 1.65 cm ($\frac{5}{8}$ in) in length. The larger seeds are preferred for confectionery purposes; smaller black seeds are used for oil extraction.

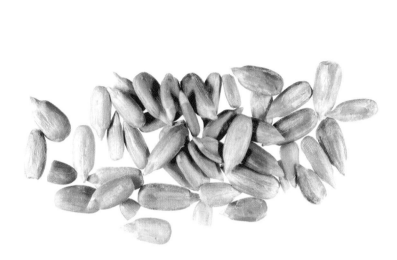

CULINARY AND NUTRITIONAL VALUE

Most sunflower seed produced is utilized for oil extraction – the rest is used for human food products and birdseed. The oil is found in salad and cooking oils, margarine, and shortenings. After extraction, the residue is included in animal feed.

Unhulled (seed coat or husk retained) seeds can be roasted and salted and sold as snack food. Hulling provides kernels, which are consumed raw or roasted, and included in salads, candies, cakes, cookies, ice-cream toppings, and spreads.

Sunflower seeds contain 27–40% polyunsaturated oil (a high percentage of linoleic acid) and 13–20% protein. In some cases, plant breeding has increased the amount of oil to 50%, and increased the percentage of monounsaturated oleic acid.

Minerals present include sodium, potassium, calcium, and iron, and the vitamins found are carotene (a small amount), the B complex, and E. Dietary fibre is present in a significant amount.

CLAIMS AND FOLKLORE

In various parts of the world, sunflower seed extracts have been used to treat lung disorders, fevers, and dysentery.

EVIDENCE

The scientific basis for the above treatments is not clear.

Sweet flag *Acorus calamus*

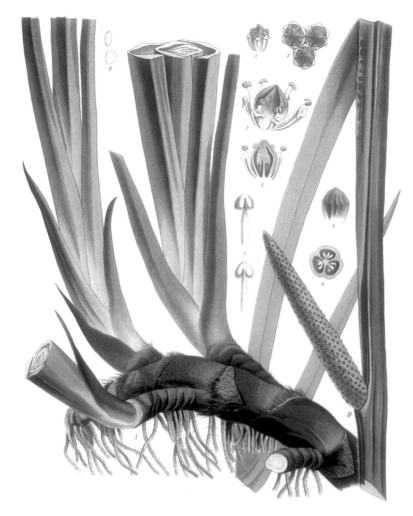

Family Araceae

ORIGIN AND CULTIVATION

Sweet flag is found all over the north temperate zone growing in wet areas such as ditches, marshy places, and the sides of lakes and rivers. At one time, it was cultivated in large quantities in the Norfolk Broads (England). The variegated forms, particularly, are grown as ornamentals. *Acorus gramineus* is known in Chinese medicine.

PLANT DESCRIPTION

Sweet flag is a semi-evergreen perennial, with a rhizome bearing lanceolate leaves, and attaining a height of between 30 cm (1 ft) and 1.5 m (5 ft). The flowers, borne on a solitary spadix, are yellow–green.

The parts of *Acorus calamus* used are the rhizome and oil.

CULINARY AND NUTRITIONAL VALUE

Extracts of the rhizome and essential oil have been used as a spice and flavouring in drinks but, because of the danger of cancer (see later), are not allowed in food in a number of countries.

CLAIMS AND FOLKLORE

Sweet flag has been used in herbal medicine for thousands of years and in many parts of the world. It has been used internally to treat digestive disorders, stimulate the appetite, and deal with arthritis, strokes, and epilepsy; externally it has been utilized for treating skin diseases.

Extracts of the rhizome and essential oil have been included in soaps, detergents, creams, lotions, perfumes, hair tonics, and antidandruff preparations.

EVIDENCE

Of its various chemical constituents, the essential oil has attracted most attention. One of the substances in the oil is asarone, which has been shown to have carcinogenic properties. The amount of essential oil in the rhizome varies from 1.5 to 3.5%, according to source; also, the amount of asarone in the oil varies from 85% down to less than 10%, according to geographical source.

Because of the above situation, some countries have legal restrictions concerning the use of sweet flag.

Sweet violet *Viola odorata;* heartsease *V. tricolor*

Family Violaceae

ORIGIN AND CULTIVATION

- Sweet violet is found on banks, under hedges, and in woods over much of Europe and Asia.

- Heartsease occurs on hilly pastures and banks, in cultivated and waste places throughout Europe, temperate Asia, and North Africa, and is naturalized in the Americas.

PLANT DESCRIPTION

- Sweet violet is a perennial with long runners and ovate to heart-shaped leaves. Its flowers are dark purple or white. The plant grows to a height of about 15 cm (6 in).

- Heartsease is an annual, biennial, or short-lived perennial with oblong to heart-shaped leaves. The flowers are purple, whitish, or yellow with a mixture of these colours. It grows to a height of about 38 cm (15 in).

All parts of both species may be utilized in herbal medicine.

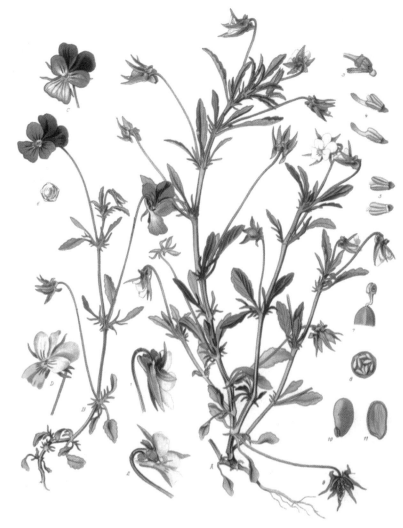

CULINARY AND NUTRITIONAL VALUE

The flowers of sweet violet are used to flavour and colour confectionery, and are included in breath fresheners.

CLAIMS AND FOLKLORE

- Sweet violet has been used to treat bronchial and respiratory catarrh, coughs, asthma, and cancer of the breast, lungs, and digestive tract.

  The oil of sweet violet, or its synthetic equivalent, is used in perfumery.

- Heartsease is supposed to be useful in treating a variety of complaints such as bronchitis, whooping cough, rheumatism, and skin and urinary problems.

EVIDENCE

A variety of chemical substances have been identified, including flavonoids in both sweet violet and heartsease, but it has not been possible to find any clinical or scientific studies relating to the efficacy of the two species.

  V. tricolor is approved in Germany, but not *V. odorata*.

Tea tree *Melaleuca alternifolia*

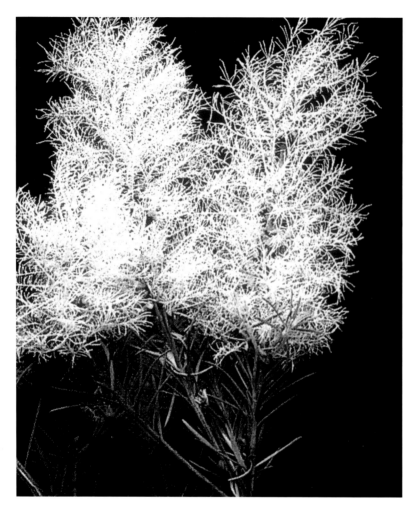

Family Myrtaceae

ORIGIN AND CULTIVATION

From the fresh leaves and twigs of *Melaleuca alternifolia* is produced the essential oil – tea tree oil – by steam distillation. The oil has powerful antiseptic properties. *M. alternifolia* and related species have been used medicinally by the Aborigines of Australia. It is reputed that members of the crews of Captain James Cook's expeditions in the late 1700s were the first Europeans to become aware of the medicinal value of the plant. Tea tree oil was used by the Australian forces in the Second World War for dressing wounds.

M. alternifolia flourishes in moist soils in New South Wales and Queensland, and there is cultivation, especially in New South Wales.

A number of other *Melaleuca* species produce essential oils of medicinal value. One of the best known is *M. leucadendron*, the source of cajaput oil.

PLANT DESCRIPTION

M. alternifolia is a shrub or small tree, 5–7 m (23 ft) in height, with a papery bark, and pointed leaves up to 3.5 cm ($1\frac{1}{2}$ in) long. In spring, small white flowers are produced in dense spikes up to 5 cm (2 in) in length. These give rise to tiny woody capsules.

CULINARY AND NUTRITIONAL VALUE
None.

CLAIMS AND FOLKLORE

Tea tree oil is strongly antiseptic, and is said to be antibacterial, antifungal, and possibly antiviral. Its main uses are for dealing with skin complaints such as burns, sunburn, acne, cold sores, boils, thrush, and vaginal infections. In such cases it would be diluted with a carrier oil (e.g. almond). It has been suggested that it could be applied directly to verrucas and warts, and to treat head lice. The oil seems to be non-toxic, and has been used in deodorants, soaps, mouthwashes, and toilet waters. There have been claims that it could give topical temporary relief for muscle and joint pains.

It has also been suggested that tea tree might be taken internally for certain ailments. This suggestion should be treated with great caution.

EVIDENCE

Tea tree oil contains a number of constituents, including terpinen-4-ol, which is antiseptic, and cineole, which is a skin irritant. In 1985 a quality standard for tea tree oil was established in Australia that called for the oil to contain 30% or more terpinen-4-ol and less than 15% cineole. The higher quality oils have 40–7% terpinen-4-ol and 2.5% cineole. A high terpinen-4-ol to low cineole ratio is best for predictable clinical results.

A number of scientific investigations have supported the antiseptic value of the oil. One interesting suggestion is that it effectively kills antibiotic-resistant 'Golden Staph' (methicillin-resistant *Staphylococcus aureus*).

Thuja, arbor-vitae *Thuja occidentalis*

Family Cupressaceae

ORIGIN AND CULTIVATION
Thuja is an evergreen tree native to northeastern North America; it grows in moist places, such as banks of streams and rivers. It is cultivated as an ornamental in Europe. Thuja is a member of the gymnosperms; i.e. the seed is exposed, not enclosed in fruit as in the flowering plants (angiosperms). *Thuja occidentalis* has been used in Chinese medicine.

PLANT DESCRIPTION
The tree may grow to a height of 20 m (65 ft). Its bark is orange–brown, the leaves are scale-like, and the greenish yellow flowers give rise to cones that are brown when ripe, about 1 cm ($\frac{3}{8}$ in) in length.

The leaves are used to prepare herbal medicine.

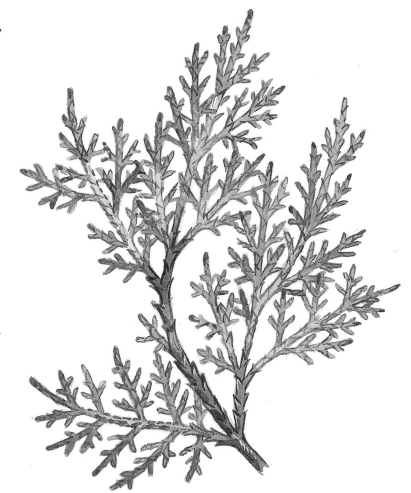

CULINARY AND NUTRITIONAL VALUE
Its essential oil may be used as a flavour ingredient in food.

CLAIMS AND FOLKLORE
Extracts are said to be antiviral and antifungal, and have been used to treat various skin diseases, including warts and polyps. Thuja has expectorant properties, so that it has been given for catarrh, bronchitis, and other respiratory complaints. It has also been used as an emmenagogue (to stimulate menstruation). In addition, thuja has served as a counter-irritant when applied to painful joints. In Germany it has been given as a non-specific immunostimulant. It may be a fragrance ingredient in soaps, creams, and similar products.

EVIDENCE
The active principle in thuja is the essential oil (containing up to 60% thujone). It has not been possible to locate any scientific investigations, but it is clear that an excess of the drug can be toxic. Therefore, it should only be used under professional supervision, and should not be given during pregnancy and lactation.

Uva-ursi, bearberry *Arctostaphylos uva-ursi*

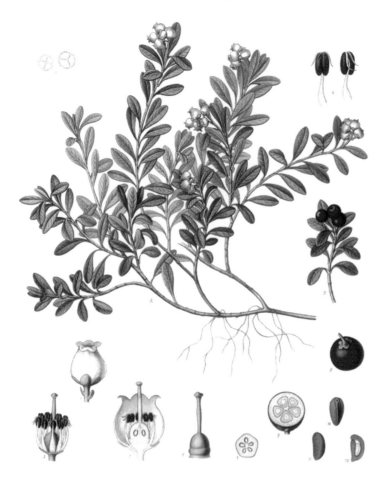

Family Ericaceae

ORIGIN AND CULTIVATION

Although originating in Europe, the plant is now found throughout the Northern Hemisphere. It grows in heathland and grassland. The major producing country is Spain.

PLANT DESCRIPTION

Uva-ursi is a low growing, up to 50 cm (20 in) in height, evergreen shrub with obovate leaves and pink flowers that give rise to red berries.

Herbal medicine is made from the leaves.

CULINARY AND NUTRITIONAL VALUE

None.

CLAIMS AND FOLKLORE

It is said to have astringent, diuretic, and urinary antiseptic properties. The drug has been used to combat bacterial infection of the urinary tract in conditions such as cystitis and urethritis.

Uva-ursi was first recorded in a Welsh thirteenth-century herbal.

EVIDENCE

Animal and human studies seem to support the claimed urinary antiseptic action of uva-ursi, although more clinical studies would be welcome. Its chemical constituents include flavonoids, tannins, and a hydroquinone derivative known as arbutin, which is regarded as the active antibacterial agent. The herb seems only to be effective as a urinary antiseptic in an alkaline medium; therefore, patients should avoid acidic fruits and their juices.

Too large a dose of the drug can lead to ringing in the ears, vomiting, delirium, convulsions, and even death. The large quantity of tannin (15–20%) in the leaf can lead to stomach disorders, so that if the medicine is prepared directly from the leaf, cold water is recommended as the extraction medium and then for 12–24 hours.

Uva-ursi should not be given to those with kidney disorders or to children, and should not be used during pregnancy and lactation.

There is support in Germany for the herb as a mild urinary antiseptic.

Uva-ursi is a member of the family Ericaceae, as is cranberry; it has also been claimed that cranberry is a urinary antiseptic, although, in its case, the fruits, not the leaves, are the source of herbal medicine.

Valerian *Valeriana officinalis*

Family Valerianaceae

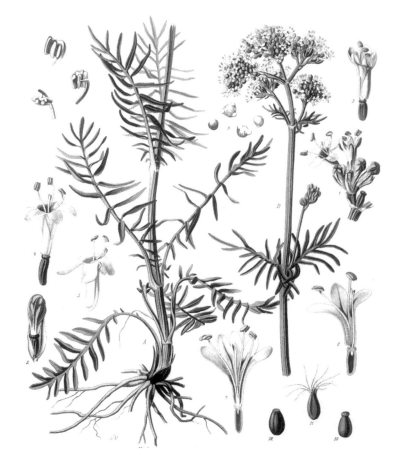

ORIGIN AND CULTIVATION
Valeriana officinalis (the common valerian) is native to Eurasia and naturalized in North America. Major producers include Belgium, France, and the former USSR. India is the major producer of Indian valerian (*V. jatamansii* syn. *V. walchii*). On a world basis there are a considerable number of other valerian species, some of which are used for herbal medicine.

PLANT DESCRIPTION
V. officinalis is an herbaceous perennial growing to a height of up to 1.5 m (5 ft). The erect and hollow stem bears deeply dissected leaves, each with 7–10 pairs of lance-shaped leaflets, and there is a terminal inflorescence of small pinkish white flowers.

Indian valerian is a smaller plant, growing to a height of about 70 cm (2 ft).

The drug is derived from the underground parts of the plant – rhizomes, stolons, and roots – although it is usually described as valerian root.

CULINARY AND NUTRITIONAL VALUE
Extracts and the essential oil of the common valerian are used as flavour components (forming up to 0.01% of the commodity) in many major food products, e.g. beer and other alcoholic drinks, non-alcoholic root beer, frozen dairy desserts, meat products, and confectionery. It is said to be especially important in apple flavours.

CLAIMS AND FOLKLORE
Valerian root has been used as a herbal drug for thousands of years – Hippocrates used it in the fourth century BC and it was described in Anglo-Saxon herbals.

Its main functions have been as a sedative and tranquillizer to treat migraine, insomnia, hysteria, fatigue, and other nervous conditions, it is also said to have antispasmodic, carminative, and stomachic properties. In the First World War the tincture was used to alleviate shell shock.

Extracts of valerian root have been applied externally for sores, eczema, and pimples. The oil has been used as a bait for trapping wild cats and rodents. Valerian root is available in herbal teas, tinctures, capsules, and tablets.

The development in fairly recent times of drugs such as barbiturates has led to a decrease in the use of valerian.

EVIDENCE
Among the chemicals present in valerian root are (a) an essential oil (containing monoterpenes and sesquiterpenes), and (b) valepotriates (iridoids). There is no doubt from human and animal experiments that valerian can act as a mild sedative, but the actual chemical mechanism is not fully understood – it is probably the result of interaction between the various constituents. Valepotriates, if stored for too long, can undergo decomposition. It is supported in Germany as a mild tranquillizer.

Valerian is generally non-toxic, but it is recommended that it should not be used during pregnancy or taken with alcohol.

Vitamin, mineral, and trace element supplements

There is a huge range of vitamin and mineral supplements now available. These may take the form of individual vitamins or mixtures of several vitamins, with or without minerals added, designed for specific age groups or for different purposes. For example, they may have different amounts of certain vitamins if they are designed for menopausal women, or for the elderly, or for children.

The orthodox nutritionist's viewpoint is that it is better to obtain the necessary vitamins and minerals by eating a variety of foods as part as a balanced diet. The discovery of substances in foods that are not strictly nutrients supports this view, as these would not previously have been included in nutrient supplements. Now, of course, supplements are being produced with bioflavonoids or polyphenols added – but the same issue arises: are there other substances in food that are biologically active that we still do not know about, which may have benefits alone or by acting synergistically with other food components to maintain health?

The requirements for vitamins (and minerals) are the subject of much deliberation by expert committees, and guidelines are given for the amounts needed in the diet to maintain health. However, there are those who consider that this is not sufficient, and that busy, stressful lives require the consumption of supplements in order to achieve 'optimum' nutrition. There is also the idea that 'processed foods' are lower in nutrients than fresh foods. While there are arguments for and against each of these viewpoints, what may be true is that people are not always able, for one reason or another, to eat an ideal 'balanced' diet. In this case the consumption of a multivitamin (with or without mineral supplements) may act as an 'insurance policy' to ensure adequate micronutrient intake. If you feel the need for a supplement the best type to choose is one that provides about 100% of the recommended dietary amount (recommended nutrient intake in the UK, recommended daily allowances in the USA) of the known vitamins, minerals, and trace elements. By doing this you can be reasonably sure that you will not be overdosing on any of those that are potentially harmful in large amounts.

Groups for whom specific vitamin supplements may be necessary are:

Breast-fed infants	A and D
Children 1–5 years	A and D
Women, pre-pregnancy	Folic acid
Pregnant women	Folic acid, D
Older people (over 65)	B_{12}
Smokers	C
Those not exposed to the sun	D
People at risk of osteoporosis	D
People on restricted diets	Multivitamins

There are also some vitamins for which a special case can be made for supplementation in specific situations, and these are described below. For information on the roles, sources, and requirements for vitamins, see the Introduction (p. xxii), and for an extensive review of dietary supplements and their use see the Recommended reading section.

VITAMIN B₆: PYRIDOXINE

Vitamin B_6 is a water-soluble vitamin with functions in various body systems. The active metabolite is involved in the metabolism of several other vitamins and in the production of haemoglobin (the oxygen-carrying pigment in blood), and is also important in the synthesis of several neurotransmitters.

The requirement for vitamin B_6 is related to protein intake (in the UK the recommended nutrient intake for adults is 15 µg per gram of protein per day). Frank deficiency disease is rare, but if deficiency does occur (e.g. in alcoholics or through drug–nutrient interaction) a range of symptoms such as dermatitis, sore mouth, sore tongue, and angular stomatitis (cracks at the corner of the mouth) may occur.

There are several disorders where, when low B_6 status has been confirmed by blood tests, supplementation with the vitamin has been shown to be beneficial. However, in these same disorders no benefit is seen if there is no evidence of low vitamin status. Conditions where this is the case are: idiopathic carpal tunnel syndrome, where compression of the median nerve in the wrist causes pain and numbness; adult asthma (where low B_6 status may be related to treatment with theophylline); and neuropathy in diabetic patients. In all of these situations the doses used have been much higher than would be possible by dietary means (10–500 times the recommended nutrient intake), and it is advisable to seek medical advice before consuming such large amounts.

The potential benefits of vitamin B_6 in premenstrual syndrome have been extensively studied in recent years. Large doses (500–800 mg per day) have been advocated, and have been shown to be effective in alleviating symptoms, but at these doses the potential for adverse side-effects is a cause for concern. Recent studies have shown benefit from much lower doses, i.e. about 50 mg per day.

At high doses the potential side-effects include peripheral neuropathy, numbness and tingling in the feet and hands, unsteady gait, loss of tendon reflexes, photosensitivity in sunlight, dizziness, nausea, breast tenderness, and exacerbation of acne.

Vitamin, mineral, and trace element supplements

In the UK the Committee on Toxicity of Chemicals in Food, Consumer Products and the Environment concluded that toxic effects can occur in doses above 50 mg per day, and the Department of Health now recommends a daily intake of not more than 10 mg per day. The US National Academy of Sciences recommend an upper limit of 100 mg per day.

FOLIC ACID

Folic acid is the parent molecule for a range of substances generally called folates. Folic acid is not found naturally in foods, but is very stable and is used to fortify foods (such as breakfast cereals). Mixtures of folates are found in foods but their bioavailability is variable. The vitamin is essential in cell division, particularly in rapidly dividing cells.

Symptoms and signs of deficiency include megaloblastic anaemia, weakness, tiredness, irritability, forgetfulness, breathlessness, anorexia, diarrhoea, headache, fainting, palpitations, and a sore tongue. The recommended nutrient intake for folate for non-pregnant adults in the UK is 200 μg per day. The 1990 Survey of British Adults showed that women consumed, on average, about 220 μg and men 312 μg per day, but that about 4% of women of child-bearing age were consuming intakes at a level at which deficiency of the vitamin is likely.

Low folate status has been implicated in two major health problems. It has been demonstrated that women with low folate status at the time of conception and during the first 12 weeks of pregnancy are more likely to have a child with a neural-tube defect (spina bifida). Women who are planning to become pregnant are advised to take an extra 400 μg of folic acid per day, i.e. a total of 600 μg per day prior to and for the first 12 weeks of pregnancy. It is difficult to obtain this amount from food, and supplements are therefore advised.

It has also been suggested that low folate status increases the risk of coronary heart disease. High levels of the amino acid homocysteine in the blood are a known risk marker for coronary heart disease (and may possibly be implicated in stroke and diabetes), and low folate intake has been shown to be related to high homocysteine levels. Supplementation with folic acid has shown mixed results in lowering homocysteine levels, and some scientists think that vitamin B_{12} intake may also be important. Research is still under way to examine whether increasing folate status can prevent coronary heart disease, but in the USA folic acid is added to flour, and this is currently being investigated in the UK.

Folic acid does not appear to have any adverse effects per se, but consumption of the vitamin may mask the effects of megaloblastic anaemia caused by vitamin B_{12} deficiency.

VITAMIN C

Vitamin C is a water-soluble vitamin otherwise known as ascorbic acid. Vitamin C is found in plant foods and is sensitive to oxygen, being oxidized to an inactive form as soon as the fruit or vegetable is cut. In cooking the vitamin is leached out into the water – using vegetable water to make sauce or gravy retains the vitamin. The recommended intake in the UK is 40 mg per day for adults (and 75 mg per day in the USA).

Vitamin C is essential for formation of collagen, and helps maintain the integrity of skin, bone, and teeth, as well as blood capillaries. It acts as an antioxidant, reacting with water-soluble free radicals, and aids in the absorption of iron from non-animal sources. It is also essential in the metabolism of folic acid and various amino acids.

Deficiency of vitamin C results in scurvy, which is now rare. Subclinical deficiency may be associated with poor wound healing and ulceration. Early signs of deficiency may be non-specific, and include lethargy, weakness, fatigue, shortness of breath, and aching limbs. Petechiae (tiny bruises) appear as deficiency advances, and bleeding around hair follicles, gums, and joints develops.

Taking megadoses of Vitamin C has been said to confer various benefits, ranging from prevention of colds, through benefits in wound healing, to prevention of heart disease and cancer. Many of the links between vitamin C and disease prevention are epidemiological, and relate to the observations that populations consuming good sources such as fruit and vegetables have a lower incidence of certain diseases. However, it is difficult to tease out the contribution of vitamin C per se when these foods contain other biologically active compounds such as beta-carotene and folate. Following the advice to eat five portions of fruit and vegetables per day will give all the biologically active compounds rather than a single vitamin.

Prevention of the common cold

Many studies have examined Linus Pauling's suggestion that very large doses (1–2 g or more per day) of vitamin C will prevent or alleviate the common cold. The evidence for an effect has been equivocal: some studies show benefit but many do not, and a recent meta-analysis concluded that there is no evidence that vitamin C prevents colds, although it may reduce the duration of symptoms.

Vitamin, mineral, and trace element supplements

Wound healing

Studies of surgical patients showed accelerated rates of wound healing when vitamin C supplements were given. In patients with pressure sores faster healing was seen after 1 month when patients were given 1 g of the vitamin daily.

Prevention of cataracts

As cataracts develop the vitamin C content of the lens of the eye declines, and patients with cataracts have been found to have lower intakes of the vitamin than those without cataracts. This does not necessarily support supplementation with large doses of the vitamin, but suggests that adequate intake is important.

Prevention of cancer

Vitamin C is an antioxidant, and may enhance the immune system as well as blocking the formation of potential carcinogens from compounds in the food or water. Studies on the potential for prevention of cancer are inconclusive for lung, breast, colon, and rectum, but there is stronger evidence of a protective effect for stomach cancer.

Prevention of coronary heart disease

The evidence for a role of vitamin C in the prevention of heart disease is not unequivocal. Some studies suggest there is a link between low intakes and heart disease, but others do not. High doses of vitamin C have been shown to reduce blood cholesterol in young people but not in older age groups. There is some evidence that people with higher intakes of the vitamin have lower blood pressure.

Contraindications

Intakes of more than 1 g of vitamin C per day may cause diarrhoea, and also increase the risk of oxalate stone formation in the kidneys, and are therefore not considered advisable. Prolonged consumption of megadoses of vitamin C (e.g. 500–1000 mg per day) increases the turnover of the vitamin in the body, and if stopped suddenly may result in rebound scurvy. People who choose to take supplements at this level should not take them for more than a few weeks, and should gradually reduce the dose rather than stopping abruptly.

ANTIOXIDANT VITAMINS

Vitamins A (in the form of beta-carotene), C, and E are sometimes referred to as the 'antioxidant vitamins' and may be sold together as such. Supplements of A, C, and E together with the trace element selenium are also available.

These, together with other food components, act to prevent damage caused by free radicals produced by various essential body functions (see p. xxv). Vitamin C is water soluble and found in aqueous solution throughout the body. Vitamin E and beta-carotene are fat-soluble vitamins that exist in lipoproteins and cell membranes; these membranes contain fats (lipids) that are particularly vulnerable to oxidative stress, and the antioxidant vitamins help prevent this.

There is growing evidence that free-radical damage is implicated in the development of many diseases, including atherosclerosis, some cancers, Parkinson's and other neurodegenerative diseases, inflammatory bowel diseases, and lung disease. However, there is little evidence to suggest that supplementation of adequately nourished people with antioxidant vitamins will reduce the incidence of the above diseases. Studies show that people with adequate blood levels of vitamin E, beta-carotene, and vitamin C are less likely to develop coronary heart disease and certain cancers. Epidemiological data from two large studies carried out on health professionals in the USA suggested that women who took more than 200 units and men who took more than 100 units of vitamin E per day had a lower incidence of coronary heart disease. (A unit of vitamin E is equivalent to 1mg of alpha tocopherol acetate. Vitamin E units are no longer officially used in the UK, but the term may be used by supplement manufacturers.) There was also a suggestion that supplementation with 50mg of beta-carotene on alternate days resulted in fewer heart attacks in men who had angina. Studies using antioxidant supplements in patients with various cancers have not produced unequivocal benefits, but it may be that these vitamins are protective against the early stages of cancer development.

Many of the studies investigating the role of antioxidant vitamins show that people with high intakes of vegetables and fruit have a lower incidence of coronary heart disease and certain cancers, and suggest that the antioxidant vitamins in these foods may be the active agents. It would seem that the best way of obtaining these vitamins is to eat a variety of fruits and vegetables each day – the UK guidelines of five portions per day (equivalent to the 450 g per day advised by the World Health Organization) is a sensible level to aim for. Antioxidant supplements commonly contain doses of vitamins C and E that are up to 10 times the recommended daily amounts (there are no recommended daily allowances for carotene), and it is probably wise to select one with moderate vitamin content as there have been studies where potentially harmful effects have been seen.

Vitamin, mineral, and trace element supplements

MINERAL AND TRACE ELEMENT SUPPLEMENTS

As with vitamins, it is considered to be best to obtain our mineral requirements from food. Information about all the important minerals and trace elements is given on pp. xviii–xxii. As with vitamins, if you wish to take supplements it is best not to exceed the recommended nutrient intake or recommended daily allowances – and care must be taken regarding the combinations taken as high doses of certain minerals can affect the absorption of others. Some further information is given below about some of the minerals and trace elements that are commonly seen as supplements.

Iron

In the UK the average adult intakes of dietary iron are adequate, but there are some groups in the population who do not obtain enough iron in the diet. The main groups at risk of low iron intake are:

- infants and children from the age of 6 months to 2 years
- younger adolescents (especially girls)
- women of child-bearing age
- pregnant women
- vegetarians.

Iron deficiency results in a type of anaemia where the red blood cells are smaller and paler than usual and are less able to carry oxygen to the body tissues. Symptoms include tiredness, weakness, pale skin, breathlessness on exertion, and sometimes palpitations. People with severe iron deficiency have impaired intellectual performance, poor work capacity, and poor immune and nerve functions. In children low iron status may affect learning ability and behaviour.

It is preferable to obtain the necessary iron from food sources (see Introduction) but supplements may be useful in some situations. (Babies and toddlers should obtain all the iron they need without supplements provided that appropriate milk formula are used. Consult a Health Visitor or dietitian for advice about appropriate formulae.) Iron is toxic at doses of 40 mg or more per day in adults, and the maximum daily supplement dose in the UK is recommended to be not more than 4 mg. Care should be taken as supplements are available that contain up to 50 mg. Iron supplements may be in liquid or tablet form. Liquid supplements should be diluted well and taken through a straw (to prevent discoloration of the teeth). Iron is best taken on an empty stomach to maximize absorption, but if taken with food there is less risk of stomach upsets.

Iron supplements may cause gastrointestinal irritation, nausea, and constipation, which can be a particular problem in the elderly. Routine iron supplementation is no longer the rule in pregnancy; iron status should be monitored and supplements taken only on advice from an appropriate health professional.

Absorption of iron may be affected by various drugs, including antacids, some antibiotics, and other nutrient supplements. Calcium supplements may reduce iron absorption; large doses of iron may reduce absorption of copper and zinc, and vice versa, and iron reduces absorption of manganese. Vitamin E requirements may be increased if large doses of iron supplements are taken, and vitamin E supplements may prevent adequate blood-forming responses in people with iron deficiency anaemia.

For all the above reasons it is probably best to take advice from a health professional if you are contemplating taking iron supplements. This is always advisable in the case of infants and young children.

Zinc

Zinc is a trace element that occurs naturally in a variety of foods (see Introduction, p. xx). In the UK diet the average intakes are slightly above the daily recommended nutrient intakes, which implies that there are individuals who have lower intakes.

Zinc deficiency may cause a variety of problems. Mild to moderate deficiency may result in poor appetite, rough skin, mental lethargy, delayed wound healing, impaired sense of taste, growth retardation, and male hypogonadism. Severe deficiency may result in diarrhoea, dermatitis, alopecia (hair loss resulting in baldness), weight loss, psychiatric disorders, and susceptibility to infection (due to impaired immune function), as well as the previously mentioned problems. Maternal zinc deficiency prior to and during pregnancy may lead to poor fetal growth and congenital malformations in the fetus.

Zinc is present in both animal and plant foods; it is best absorbed when associated with certain amino acids (e.g. cystine and histidine), so it is well absorbed from meat, fish, and dairy products. The zinc in plant foods such as wholegrain cereals (especially bran products) and soya protein is less well absorbed. However, the zinc content of wholegrain foods is higher than in more refined products, and this may compensate for the absorptive effects.

The absorption of zinc may be reduced by oral iron supplements (and vice versa) and by folic acid. These effects could be of concern in pregnant women, who may be advised to take iron and folic acid.

Vitamin, mineral, and trace element supplements

People take zinc supplements for a variety of reasons. There is little evidence that extra zinc is useful in treating acne or the common cold. Zinc supplements have been shown to promote wound healing in people with initially low zinc levels, but not in those whose zinc status is adequate. Healing appears to be more rapid in some types of leg ulcers if patients are given zinc supplements.

It has been suggested that zinc deficiency may be involved in the development of anorexia nervosa. If food intake is restricted during the period of rapid growth at puberty, zinc deficiency might precipitate anorexia. Studies have shown short- and long-term benefits for doses of about 45 mg per day in promoting weight gain in young women with anorexia nervosa, but medical advice should be sought in these circumstances.

Doses of zinc in excess of 50 mg per day over a prolonged period may have deleterious effects; doses over 150 mg per day may result in depressed immune function, stomach problems, and abnormal blood lipid levels, while acute toxicity, with diarrhoea, nausea, and vomiting, may occur at a dose of 200 mg.

Selenium

Selenium is a trace element that acts as an antioxidant, protecting the polyunsaturated fats in cell membranes from damage by free radicals (see p. xxv). Selenium is found in foods from both plants and animals. The richest sources of selenium are fish (tuna fish is an excellent source) and brazil nuts. Mushrooms are a good source but the selenium content of plant foods depends very much on the soil in which the crop is grown. Until recently, in the UK, bread was the most important contributor to the selenium content of the diet, as it was made from hard North American wheat that was rich in the trace element. However, in the last 15 years or so the North American wheat has been replaced by softer, home-grown wheat that has a lower content of selenium, and hence bread has become a much less important source. In most diets meat and dairy products are now the main sources, and it is possible that vegetarians (especially vegans) may have low intakes.

Some epidemiological studies have suggested that low intakes of selenium may be associated with higher incidence of cancers, especially of the gut and respiratory tract, but as yet there is no confirmation of this. The potential role for selenium in the prevention of heart disease is also unclear at present, and there is no proven benefit for selenium in treating arthritis or hair and nail problems.

Selenium is toxic if taken in excess. Symptoms include hair loss, nail changes, skin lesions, diarrhoea, nausea, tiredness, and peripheral nerve damage. There is a very narrow margin between the safe and toxic levels of selenium. Doses of between 50 and 100 μg are safe, but the intake from all sources should not exceed 450 μg per day. It is suggested that the maximum dose from supplements should not exceed 200 μg per day. Selenium is often sold in combination with the antioxidant vitamins A, C, and E.

White bryony   *Bryonia dioica*

Family Cucurbitaceae

ORIGIN AND CULTIVATION

Bryonia dioica is quite common in hedges and woods in central and southern Europe. *B. alba* is used in homeopathic medicine.

PLANT DESCRIPTION

It is a climbing perennial plant that can grow to a great height. The leaves are divided into five or seven lobes and there are tendrils for climbing. Plants are male or female. Red or orange berries are produced. There is a thick, tuberous rootstock or root.

Herbal medicine is prepared from the rootstock.

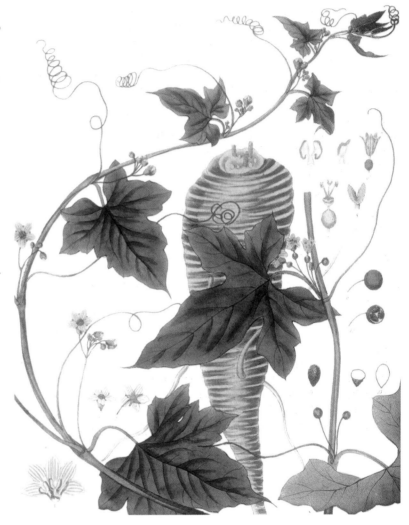

CULINARY AND NUTRITIONAL VALUE

None.

CLAIMS AND FOLKLORE

It is reputed that Dioscorides used the plant for herbal medicine, and it was employed in medieval Britain to treat leprosy.

The herb is bitter and a strong purgative. Extracts are given internally for inflammatory conditions such as rheumatism, arthritis, asthma, and bronchitis, and to reduce hypertension. Externally, it has been applied as a counter-irritant and rubefacient to painful joints.

EVIDENCE

White bryony contains cucurbitacins (bitter compounds), glycosides, essential oils, and tannins. The herb is not used much today and great care should be taken because an excess can be toxic. It should not be given during pregnancy and lactation. The herb is not approved in Germany.

White willow *Salix alba and other species*

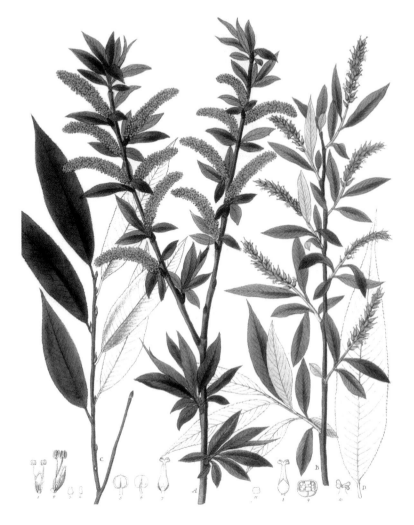

Family Salicaceae

ORIGIN AND CULTIVATION
Willow species are shrubs or trees found throughout the temperate and cold regions of the Northern Hemisphere. They often appreciate damp places such as river banks.

PLANT DESCRIPTION
Salix alba can grow to a height of 25 m (82 ft). It is deciduous, with brown bark, and lanceolate leaves, up to 10 cm (4 in) in length. The flowers are found in catkins.

The bark is the source of the herbal drug. The leaves have also been used, but to a lesser extent.

CULINARY AND NUTRITIONAL VALUE
None.

CLAIMS AND FOLKLORE
Dioscorides (first century) suggested the leaves as a means of relieving back pain. Native North Americans used bark tea to bring about sweating to reduce fever.

Willow has been employed as an anti-inflammatory drug for rheumatism and arthritis in the back and joints; it has also been used to treat headaches and fevers. Willow is astringent, and was regarded as a possible means of stopping bleeding.

EVIDENCE
Willow contains salicylates (salicylic acid), tannins, and flavonoids. Salicylic acid was first synthesized in 1838, and gave rise to the synthetic drug aspirin in 1899. The percentage of salicylates varies amongst *Salix* species, from 0.5 from 10.0%.

Apparently, relatively few experimental studies have been carried out into the value of willow; nevertheless, because it contains salicylates it is felt that, like aspirin, it can act as an analgesic and anti-inflammatory agent, thus supporting its herbal uses.

Individuals who, because of certain conditions, are hypersensitive to aspirin, should likewise avoid willow. The herbal medicine should not be taken in addition to aspirin, and any drug interactions with aspirin also apply to willow. One advantage of willow, as opposed to aspirin, is that it does not irritate the stomach.

Willow is best avoided during pregnancy and lactation. It is supported in Germany.

Wild yam, colic root *Dioscorea villosa*

Family Dioscoreaceae

ORIGIN AND CULTIVATION

Wild yam is found in the woods and thickets of the USA.

PLANT DESCRIPTION

It is a climber that may grow to a height of 5–6 m (20 ft). There is an underground slender rhizome and the heart-shaped leaves are up to 10 cm (4 in) in length. Its minute flowers are green–yellow in colour. The closely related *Dioscorea quaternata* is difficult to distinguish from *D. villosa*.

The rhizome and roots are the sources of the herbal drug.

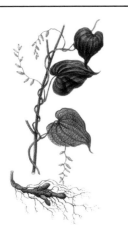

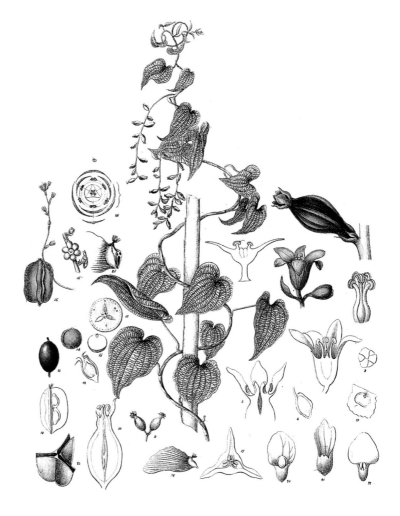

CULINARY AND NUTRITIONAL VALUE

None.

CLAIMS AND FOLKLORE

The herbal extract has been taken internally for a variety of complaints, including rheumatism, arthritis, colic, gastritis, bronchitis, and painful menstruation. This has been related to its anti-inflammatory and antispasmodic actions.

EVIDENCE

Wild yam contains steroidal saponins, alkaloids, tannins, and some other substances. Diosgenin, a steroidal saponin, was first isolated from *Dioscorea* species in 1936, and it can be converted in the laboratory into various steroidal substances such as oral contraceptives and hormones.

It has been claimed that the yam steroidal substance is the anti-inflammatory agent, although no scientific evidence has been uncovered. Also, claims that wild yam products applied externally or taken internally can lead to hormone synthesis in the body and improve various complaints have no scientific basis.

The drug should not be taken during pregnancy and lactation.

Witch hazel *Hamamelis virginiana*

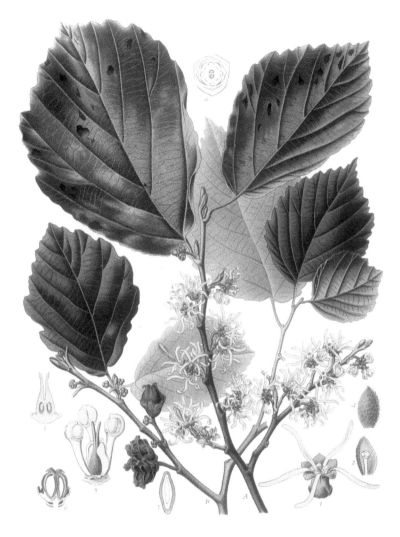

Family Hamamelidaceae

ORIGIN AND CULTIVATION
Witch hazel is a native of Canada and the USA, and found in moist woods in those countries. It is a popular ornamental plant.

PLANT DESCRIPTION
The plant is a deciduous shrub or small tree that may grow to a height of 5 m (16ft). The leaves are obovate and the bark is greyish brown. When the leaves fall in the autumn, bright yellow flowers with crinkled petals are produced. These give rise to capsules that do not ripen until the following year.

Herbal medicine is prepared from the leaves and bark.

Bottled 'witch hazel' or 'witch hazel water' is prepared by steam-distilling the twigs and then adding alcohol to the distillate. The product is often available in the home.

CULINARY AND NUTRITIONAL VALUE
None.

CLAIMS AND FOLKLORE
Native North American people used the herb and the custom was acquired by the settlers. The knowledge was then sent to Europe.

The drug has been applied externally to treat varicose veins, sprains, bruises, burns, eye and skin inflammations, and some other conditions. Internally, it has been used for diarrhoea, colitis, and excessive menstruation, in addition to other complaints.

EVIDENCE
Witch hazel contains tannins, flavonoids, essential oils, and some other constituents. The drug is astringent and can check bleeding. It also seems to have some anti-inflammatory action. These actions are usually related to the high content of tannins.

There is some dispute about the effectiveness of 'witch hazel water', which does not contain tannins. It is astringent, but this could be due to the added alcohol or maybe some constituent of witch hazel. There is support in Germany for the action of the drug on some skin complaints.

It is generally regarded as non-toxic but excessive ingestion should be avoided.

Yarrow *Achillea millefolium*

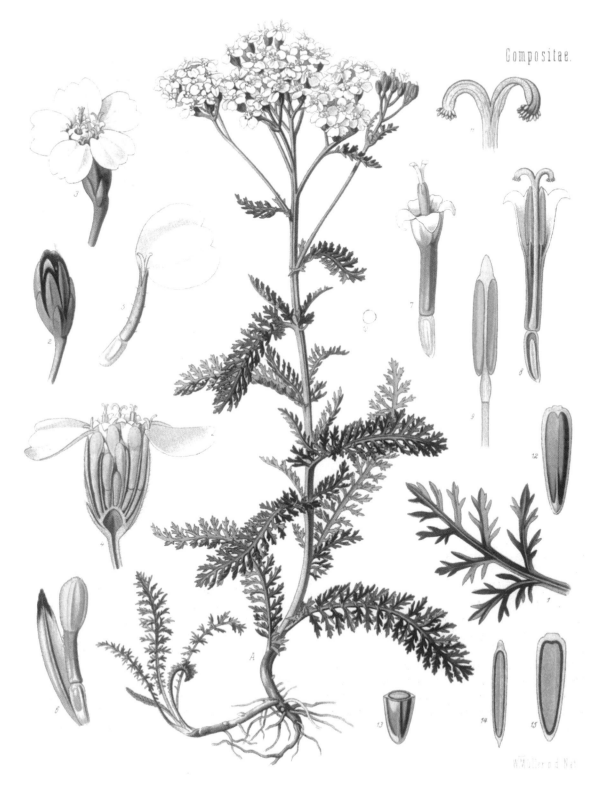

Yarrow

Family Compositae/Asteraceae

ORIGIN AND CULTIVATION

Achillea millefolium is found in Europe growing in pastures, waste places, and other locations. It is said to have been naturalized in North America, but doubt has been cast on whether the yarrow of North America is actually *A. millefolium*. Because of genetic and chemical differences, it is designated *A. lanulosa*.

A number of *Achillea* species are grown as garden ornamentals.

PLANT DESCRIPTION

Yarrow is a perennial that can grow to a height of 30 cm (1 ft). It has feathery leaves, and the flower head consists of white or pink ray florets and yellow disc florets.

The flower heads supply herbal medicine.

CULINARY AND NUTRITIONAL VALUE

In Europe, extracts of the plant can be added as a flavouring agent to food, alcoholic beverages (e.g. vermouth), and bitters, providing that the amount of thujone (a constituent of the essential oil) is regulated. In the USA it can only be added to alcoholic drinks and the final product must be thujone free.

CLAIMS AND FOLKLORE

Yarrow has a long history of being used to treat wounds, e.g. during the American Civil War. A number of properties are attributed to it. It is said to be antispasmodic, astringent, anti-inflammatory, bitter, increase sweating, act as a diuretic, stop bleeding, reduce fever, lower blood pressure, and promote menstruation. These many alleged properties have been utilized to deal with complaints such as colds, influenza, diarrhoea and other digestive problems, rheumatism, arthritis, and menstrual complaints, as well as wounds and nosebleeds.

EVIDENCE

A number of chemical compounds have been identified in the herb, including alkaloids, flavonoids, tannins, and essential oil (with many constituents such as azulene, thujone, and sesquiterpene lactones).

A number of animal experiments have been carried out. Anti-inflammatory activity is associated with the azulene component of the essential oil, which can vary from 0 to 50%. It is stated that there is no azulene in *A. millefolium*, but that it is present in *A. lanulosa* (and *A. collina*). Achilleine, an alkaloid, has been shown to reduce bleeding. Antispasmodic activity has been associated with the flavonoids. The alkaloid fraction is said to be concerned with the fever-reducing (antipyretic) activity of the herb, and the blood pressure-lowering (hypotensive) property. The tannins have an astringent action. Sesquiterpene lactones could be responsible for the bitter flavour of the herb. It is supported in Germany.

Achillea is generally non-toxic but some cases of allergy have been reported. It should not be consumed during pregnancy and lactation.

Recommended reading

Blumenthal, M., Busse, W.R., Goldberg, A., *et al.* (ed.) (1996). *German Commission E monographs: therapeutic monographs on medicinal herbs.* American Botanical Council, Austin, TX.
[An English translation of an important German work that describes some 400 herbal medicines, including their interactions, toxicities, contraindications, and dosages. About two-thirds of these are supported.]

Blumenthal, M., Goldberg, A., and Brinkmann, J. (ed.) (2000). *Herbal medicine: expanded Commission E monographs.* Integrative Medicine Communications, Newton, MA.
[An update of some of the Commission E monographs.]

Bown, D. (1995). *Encyclopedia of herbs and their uses.* Dorling Kindersley, London.
[This work covers a very wide range of herbal plants utilized in a variety of ways. The plants are well described and illustrated.]

Buttriss, J. (ed.) (2002). *Adverse reactions to food.* Blackwell Science, Oxford.
[Report on the British Nutrition Foundation Task Force. Review of the evidence for adverse reactions to foods, practical aspects of constructing diets, and a discussion of the need for further research.]

Chevallier, A. (2001). *The encyclopedia of medicinal plants* (2nd edn). Dorling Kindersley, London.
[Accounts of the utilization of a very large number of herbal plants, including dosages and methods of preparation. Profusely illustrated.]

HMSO (1989). *Dietary reference values for food energy and nutrients for the United Kingdom: report on health and social subjects 41.* HMSO, London.
[Tables of recommended nutrient intakes for the UK. Includes discussion of the derivation of the values, and reasons for the recommendations.]

Eskinazi, D. (ed.) (1999). *Botanical medicine.* Mary Ann Liebert, Larchmont, NY.
[A number of interesting chapters on the economics, trade, and legal situation of herbal plants and medicines.]

Foster, S. and Tyler, V.E. (1999). *Tyler's honest herbal* (4th edn). Haworth Press, New York.
[A description of over 100 herbs and related remedies. Their value, or lack of, is explained in very clear terms. A most useful book.]

Geissler, C.A. Powers, H.J. (eds) 2005 *Human Nutrition* (11th Edition). Elsevier, Churchill Livingstone, Edinburgh.
[Comprehensive textbook covering all aspects of nutrition and dietetics from foods through to biochemistry and clinical aspects. Detailed and well referenced.]

Gruenwald, J., Brendler, T., and Jaenicke, C. (ed.) (2000). *PDR for herbal medicines* (2nd edn). Medical Economics Company, Montvale, NJ.
[This work describes a very large number (about 700) of medicinal herbs with side-effects, interactions, and toxicities. Many photographs are included.]

Jellin, J.M., Gregory, P., Batz, F., *et al.* (ed.) (2000). *Pharmacist's letter/prescriber's letter natural medicines comprehensive database* (3rd edn). Therapeutic Research Facility, Stockton, CA.
[A very large number of herbal medicines and other materials such as foods are described, with reference to interactions, dosages, and toxicities.]

Kruger, A. (1997). *The pocket guide to herbs.* Parkgate Books, London.
[A concise account of a considerable number of herbs. Well illustrated.]

Lawrence review of natural products. Facts and Comparisons, St Louis, MO.
[An ongoing series of monographs on natural products, including health foods and herbals, covering their descriptions, chemistry, toxicology, and other aspects. Many are periodically updated and revised. A very useful series.]

Leung, A.Y. and Foster, S. (1996). *Encyclopaedia of common natural ingredients used in food, drugs and cosmetics* (2nd edn). John Wiley, New York.
[As the book name indicates, this work describes a large number of natural ingredients and their utilization in food, health foods, and medicine.]

Macrae, R., Robinson, R.K., and Sadler, M.J. (ed.) (1993). *Encyclopaedia of food science, food technology and nutrition,* Vols 1–8. Academic Press, London.
[An important account of all aspects of food science and nutrition, produced by many experts.]

Mason, P. (1995). *Handbook of dietary supplements.* Blackwell Science, Oxford.
[Detailed description of a wide range of dietary supplements and the scientific evidence for their usefulness.]

Recommended reading

Mills, S. and Bone, K. (2000). *Principles and practice of phytotherapy*. Churchill Livingstone, Edinburgh.
[An impressive overview of herbal plants, and detailed accounts of about 50 species.]

National Research Council (1989). *Recommended dietary allowances* (10th edn). Subcommittee on the 10th edn of the RDAs, Food and Nutrition Board, Commission of Life Sciences, National Research Council, Washington, DC. [Tables of recommended nutrient intakes for the USA. Includes discussion of the derivation of the values and reasons for the recommendations.]

Newell, C.A., Anderson, L.A., and Phillipson, J.D. (1996). *Herbal medicines*. Pharmaceutical Press, London. [Accounts of about 100 herbal medicines, with information concerning their utilization, scientific and clinical studies, dosages, toxicities, interactions, and other relevant aspects. A very valuable addition to the herbal literature.]

Rosengarten, F. (1984). *The book of edible nuts*. Walker, New York.
[A very readable account of the utilization of common, and some uncommon, nuts.]

Royal Society of Chemistry/MAFF (1991). *McCance and Widdowson's 'the composition of foods'* (5th edn). Royal Society of Chemistry/Ministry of Agriculture, Fisheries and Food, Cambridge. Supplements: *Cereals and cereal products* (3rd supplement to 4th edn, 1988); *Vegetables, herbs and spices* (5th supplement to 4th edn, 1991); *Fruits and nuts* (1st supplement to 5th edn, 1992); *Miscellaneous food* (4th supplement to 5th edn, 1994). [Many food analysis tables – an internationally recognized work.]

Sadler, M.J., Strain, J.J., and Caballero, B. (ed.) (2005). *The encyclopedia of human nutrition*. 2nd Edition. Elsevier, St Louis. Oxford.
[Monographs on all aspects of nutrition written by experts in each field. Covers basic and clinical aspects of nutrition.]

Vaughan, J.G. and Geissler, C.A. (1997). *The new Oxford book of food plants*. Oxford University Press, Oxford. [The origin, description, and utilization of many food plants, together with their importance in human nutrition. Fully illustrated.]

Watt, B.K. and Merrill, A.L. (1975). *Handbook of the nutritional contents of foods: US Department of Agriculture*. Dover Publications, New York.
[Food analyses are given for many types of food.]

Webb, G.P. (2002). *Nutrition: a health promotion approach* (2nd edn). Arnold, New York.
[Readable text developing themes in basic and applied nutrition.]

The books below are all reports of the Standing Committee on the Scientific Evaluation of Dietary Reference Intakes. Food and Nutrition Board, Institute of Medicine, Washington, DC. They give detailed information about the derivation of dietary reference intakes in the USA and are accessible through http://www.nal.usda.gov/fnic/etext/000105

Dietary reference intakes for calcium, phosphorus, magnesium, vitamin D and fluoride (1999).

Dietary reference intakes for thiamin, riboflavin, niacin, vitamin B_6, folate, vitamin B_{12}, pantothenic acid, biotin and choline (2000).

Dietary reference intakes for vitamin C, vitamin E, selenium and carotenoids (2000).

Dietary reference intakes for vitamin A, vitamin K, arsenic, boron, chromium, copper, iodine, iron, manganese, molybdenum, nickel, silicon, vanadium and zinc (2001).

Glossary

Abortifacient causes abortion

Acne a skin disease

Allergic reacts to certain chemicals or conditions

Alterative a substance that improves nutritional health

Alzheimer's disease involves loss of memory

Anaemia a blood disease in which there is a lack of red cells

Analgesic a pain reducer

Analogue a compound with a molecular structure closely similar to that of another, but which may behave differently

Anaphylaxis a type of shock

Angina a heart disease

Annual a plant cycle completed in 1 year

Anorexia uncontrolled loss of weight

Anorexia nervosa a psychiatric disorder in which food intake is limited

Antibacterial controls growth of or kills bacteria

Antiemetic stops vomiting

Antiflatulent controls intestinal gas

Antifungal controls growth of or kills fungi

Anti-inflammatory reduces inflammation

Antimicrobial controls growth of or kills microorganisms

Antimutagenic decreases rate of mutations

Antipyretic reduces fever

Antiseptic controls growth of or kills microorganisms

Antispasmodic reduces spasms or cramps

Antithrombotic prevents blood clotting

Antitussive relieves coughs

Antiviral controls growth of or kills viruses

Aphrodisiac stimulates sexual desire

Arthritis an inflammation of the joints

Asthma a breathing disorder

Astringent hardens and tightens skin, and delicate membranes; may control bleeding, diarrhoea

Atherosclerosis hardening of the arteries

Atopic a type of eczema

Biennial a plant cycle completed in 2 years

Bioavailability a measure of the amount of nutrient in a food available for metabolism

Bipinnate a leaf with leaflets subdivided along a central axis

Bract a type of leaf associated with a flower

Bracteole a type of leaf associated with a flower

Bronchitis an inflammatory condition affecting the bronchi

Capillary a minute blood vessel

Cardiotonic improves heart function

Cardiovascular relating to heart and blood system

Carminative relieves digestive gas and indigestion

Catarrh mucus accumulation in the head and sinuses

Choleretic induces bile flow

Cirrhosis a liver disease

Colic an abdominal pain related to the intestines or bladder

Conjunctivitis an eye condition

Contraindicated not to be taken

Coronary artery disease affects the arteries that supply the heart

Counter-irritant a superficial irritant used to relieve deep-seated pain

Cultivar a variety of a cultivated plant

Cystitis a bladder condition, most common in women

Deciduous a shrub or tree whose leaves fall in autumn

Dementia involves loss of memory and other functions

Demulcent soothes and protects body surfaces

Dermatitis a skin disease

Diabetes mellitus a disorder of carbohydrate and fat metabolism

Diabetic neuropathy damage to nerves associated with diabetes mellitus

Diaphoretic induces perspiration

Dehiscent breaks open (to release seeds)

Glossary

Diuretic increases urine production

Diverticulitis an inflammation in the large intestine

Dysentery (amoebic, bacillary) colic and dysentery induced by entamoeba (an amoeba) and bacteria

Dyspepsia indigestion

Eczema a skin disease

Efficacy the ability of a drug to deal with a condition

Emetic causes vomiting

Emmenagogue promotes menstrual flow

Emollient softens or smoothes skin

Endometriosis abnormal growth of cells lining the uterus

Enzymes biological catalysts that facilitate biochemical reactions in the body

Enzymes (digestive) break down dietary fats, proteins, and complex carbohydrates into small units that can be absorbed

Epididymitis an infection of the epididymis

Epilepsy a condition associated with fits

Evergreen a shrub or tree that appears to retain leaves

Ex vivo outside the body

Expectorant clears phlegm from throat and chest

Febrifuge reduces fever

Florets small flowers

Flower head a collection of florets, as in Compositae

Fruit a product of ovary fertilization

Gastric ulcer a stomach ulcer

Gastroenteritis an infection of the stomach and intestines often leading to diarrhoea

Gram positive/negative types of bacteria

Groat the part of a cereal grain (usually oats) remaining after the outer hull is removed

Haemorrhage bleeding

Hepatitis a liver complaint

Herpes a viral infection

Homeopathy an alternative medical treatment

Hydrolysis the addition of water

Hyperactivity overactivity

Hypercalcaemia a high level of calcium in the blood

Hypercholesterolaemic a high blood-cholesterol level

Hyperglycaemia a high blood glucose level

Hypertension high blood pressure

Hyperthyroidism excessive activity of the thyroid gland

Hypoglycaemia a too-low blood glucose level

Hypotension low blood pressure

Immunostimulant stimulates the immune system

In vitro outside the body

In vivo within the body

Incontinence inability to control urination

Involucre a collection of leaves around the flower head

Irritable bowel syndrome a disease of the gut

Ischaemic heart disease an alternative name for coronary heart disease

Lactation breast feeding

Libido desire for sexual intercourse

Lipid fat

Mastalgia pain in the chest

Megaloblastic large cells

Meta-analysis a scientific study that examines the results of several papers on a particular topic

Microcytic small cells; in iron-deficiency anaemia the red blood cells are smaller than normal

Neuralgia pain affecting nerve

Neuropathy nerve damage

Neurotransmitter a chemical that passes messages from nerves to other tissues

Node a point of the stem where a leaf is attached

Nutlet a type of fruit in Labiatae – commonly called 'seed'

Obovate a leaf shape

Obstetrics the branch of medicine dealing with pregnancy and giving birth

Oestrogenic has a similar action to the female hormone oestrogen

Osteoporosis a reduced bone mass that occurs on ageing

Glossary

Ovate a leaf shape

Palmate leaflets of a leaf arranged like the fingers of a hand

Peptic ulcer a stomach ulcer

Perennial an herbaceous or woody plant that lives from year to year

Pharyngitis an infection of the mouth cavity

Photosensitive sensitive to light

Platelet activating factor a substance released by blood cells that could lead to clotting

Pleurisy a lung disease

Premenstrual syndrome emotional and unpleasant physical reactions before menstruation

Prophylactic a treatment to ward off disease

Prostaglandins chemicals with hormonal action

Prostate a gland in the male near the bladder

Psoriasis a skin disease

Receptacle part of a flower to which other parts are attached

Rhizome an underground stem

Rootstock a vertical underground structure, partly stem and partly root

Rubefacient an agent that reddens skin

Runner an overground branch that produces a new plant at its tip

Spadix a spike bearing flowers within a spathe

Spathe a large bract enclosing a flower

Spike an unbranched, elongated flower head bearing stalkless flowers

Steroid therapy treatment with steroids

Stolon an underground branch that produces a new plant at its tip

Stomachic eases stomach pain

Systemic lupus erythematosus an inflammatory auto-immune disease

Taproot the main root

Tinnitus ringing in the ears

Topical application to the body surface

Trifoliate a leaf shape

Tripinnate a leaf shape

Tuber a swollen stem, or swollen root

Umbel an inflorescence with branches like the ribs of an umbrella

Urethritis an infection of the urethra

Vasodilator relaxes and enlarges blood vessels

Vegan diet excludes all animal products

Vegetarian diet excludes meat and fish but may include dairy products and eggs

Vermifuge a medicine that expels intestinal worms

Index

Index

Index

Index

Index

Index

Index

Index

Index

Index

Index